Nutrition, Food and Drug Interactions in Man

World Review of Nutrition and Dietetics

Vol. 43

Series Editor
Geoffrey H. Bourne, Grenada, West Indies

KARGER

S. Karger · Basel · München · Paris · London · New York · Tokyo · Sydney

Nutrition, Food and Drug Interactions in Man

Volume Editor
Gérard Debry, Nancy

33 figures and 46 tables, 1984

KARGER

S. Karger · Basel · München · Paris · London · New York · Tokyo · Sydney

World Review of Nutrition and Dietetics

Vol. 40: Nutrition Education and Modern Concepts of Food Assimilation
G.H. Bourne, Grenada, West Indies (ed.)
XII + 192 p., 36 fig., 6 tab., hard cover, 1982. ISBN 3–8055–3519–8
Vol. 41: Aspects of Human and National Nutrition
G.H. Bourne, Grenada, West Indies (ed.)
XII + 260 p., 35 fig., 61 tab., hard cover, 1983. ISBN 3–8055–3591–0
Vol. 42: Nutrients and Energy
G.H. Bourne, Grenada, West Indies (ed.)
XII + 228 p., 27 fig., 44 tab., hard cover, 1983. ISBN 3–8055–3710–7

National Library of Medicine, Cataloging in Publication
Nutrition, food and drug interactions in man/
volume editor, Gérard Debry. -- Basel; New York: Karger, 1984.
(World review of nutrition and dietetics; v. 43)
Papers presented at an international symposium held Nov. 3–5, 1982, in Paris,
and sponsored by France's Ministry of Research and Industry and others. Includes index.
1. Nutrition – drug effects – congresses 2. Drug Interactions – congresses
3. Drugs – metabolism – congresses 4. Metabolism – drug effects – congresses
I. Debry, Gérard II. France, Ministère de l'Industrie et de la Recherche III. Series
W1 WO898 v. 43 [QU 145 N9738 1982]
ISBN 3–8055–3800–6

Drug Dosage
The authors and the publisher have exerted every effort to ensure that drug selection and dosage set forth in this text are in accord with current recommendations and practice at the time of publication. However, in view of ongoing research, changes in government regulations, and the constant flow of information relating to drug therapy and drug reactions, the reader is urged to check the package insert for each drug for any change in indications and dosage and for added warnings and precautions. This is particularly important when the recommended agent is a new and/or infrequently employed drug.

Printed in Switzerland by Thür AG Offsetdruck, Pratteln
ISBN 3–8055–3800–6

Advisory Board

Contents

Conclusions

Free Communications

A. Food and Drugs

B. Drug Bioavailability and Metabolism

C. Effect of Malnutrition on Drug Pharmacokinetics

Preface

For some 10 years the relations between food, nutritional status and drugs have been increasingly investigated. Cumulative evidence emerging from these studies was reviewed in 1976 in the USA during the congress organized by the American Nutrition Foundation (NF). The communications of this congress have been collected under the supervision of *John N. Hatchcock* and *Julius Coon* and published in a monograph edited by Academic Press in 1978.

It was then time for a new meeting of investigators to be organized. For that reason, thanks to the support of the Ministry of Research and Industry, of the 'Fondation Française pour la Nutrition' (FFN), of the 'Syndicat National de l'Industrie Pharmaceutique' (SNIP) and of the 'Comité National de Coordination des Etudes et des Recherches en Nutrition et en Alimentation' (CNERNA-CNRS), an international symposium was held in Paris on November 3rd, 4th and 5th 1982.

The organizing committee wishes to extend its sincere thanks to the Ministry of Research and Industry and to all those who contributed so efficiently to the success of this congress.

The aspects of the relations between food, nutritional status and drugs are multiform. They are all within the limits of the fields of several disciplines, primarily pharmacology and human nutrition. Close collaboration between pharmacologists and nutritionists is therefore essential in research if relevant results are to be achieved. The study protocols are generally difficult to draw up and to apply. These protocols are designed for generally healthy humans so that they can be their own controls. This represents considerable experimental pressure.

The experiments have to be repeated at different dosages and under different nutritional conditions. Each experiment has to be conducted for a sufficiently long duration to exploit the results obtained in human therapy. For many experimental situations, methodologies remain to be innovated.

The reports and the communications published in this volume of the congress show that the field of drug and nutrition relations is still unclear and has not been much explored to date. They will undoubtedly foster research activities and encourage pharmacologists and nutritionists to join their competences.

G. Debry

Wld Rev. Nutr. Diet., vol. 43, pp. 1–9 (Karger, Basel 1984)

Drugs, Food and Nutrition

G. Debry

Département de Nutrition et des Maladies Métaboliques de l'Université de Nancy I et Groupe Inserm U-59, Nancy, France

Food has long represented the sustenance of man and was the sole means of treatment available against illness. Food ensured the development and the maintenance of the body, and is the source of energy necessary for physical exercise. Food also enabled one to recover health in case of denutrition.

From Food to Drug

It was progressively seen that some foods had more or less marked curative properties and that, according to the regions, some plants had specific therapeutic virtues. The notion of 'drug-food' began to take shape over the centuries. In many of the Third World countries, drug-foods, both as sustenance and as treatment, still play a major role since the economy of these countries makes it difficult to instigate or develop pharmaceutical industries, or to import adequate supplies of drugs for the whole population. In relation to the concentration of active principles in the plants, some drug-foods are considered more as food than as drug and vice versa. Therefore, a chain of consumable substances which are between food and drugs exists. Illustrative of this continuum are vitamins, which act both as nutriment and as drug. It is the same case with other micronutriments of mineral origin.

The pharmaceutical industry in developed countries first drew its inspiration from the use made of drug-foods by extracting their active principles. It moreover took into account the long experience of the natives in collecting plants with potent curative or toxic properties. These plants were considered more as drugs than as food.

Religions also recognized the effects of food on health and meditation capacity, in particular the effects of ritual fasting. The history of food and drug relations according to regions, ethnic groups, religion, magical or medical practices are long-dated and most instructive regarding the relationship of man with nature and his divinities.

Evolution of Food and Drug Relations in Modern Times

The very fast advances of pharmacology and biology over the past 50 years have resulted in the production, in large quantities, of molecules of synthesis and in the administration of drugs not only by the digestive route (enterally) as in the past, but also extradigestively (parenterally) in venous or arterial blood in the cerebrospinal fluid, subcutaneously, by the airways or even directly at the level of cells using their specific metabolic or physical sensitivities. This expansion of new therapies and the unsuspected power of their healing properties have pushed the food and drug relations into the background.

More recently, the development of increasingly accurate and specific physiological or biochemical techniques has enabled pharmacokinetic investigators to follow up the fate of drugs in the system and to discover the factors affecting their metabolism. Cumulative evidence contributed to a first explanation to two phenomena which had been observed for a long time: i.e. the variations in the effects of the same dose of drug from one individual to another (interindividual variations), and day-to-day variations in the same subject (intraindividual variations). Genetic differences, as shown by *Vesell* and co-workers [1–3], sex, and age were recognized as important causes of these interindividual variations according to the nature of the drugs. Most of the reasons for intraindividual variations are, however, unexplained.

The recent discovery of the temporal factor, i.e. change in drug effect in relation to time of administration, accounts for a number of the variations observed and implies that all the necessary precisions should be given in this respect in the protocols for pharmacological and pharmacokinetic studies. This notion is so relevant that it justifies the individualization of a new scientific activity in pharmacology, i.e. chronopharmacology.

Much progress in our knowledge and in our therapeutic means have contributed to the overseeing of the role of food and nutrition. Most certainly, manufacturers of pharmaceuticals strongly advise most drugs to be taken either at the beginning or during the course of a meal. But it was more a recommendation to prevent possible intolerances or unwanted side effects such as hypoglycemia than a decision based on food and drug relations. Likewise, physicians never cared whether the same dose of a drug could be prescribed if the patient was under satisfactory nutritional conditions, was obese, or was suffering from denutrition.

Evidence of more or less severe unwanted reactions appearing when some drugs and food are ingested simultaneously, such as for instance monoamine oxidase inhibitors and cheese, or alcohol and hypoglycemic sulfonamides or hypnotics, have drawn attention to drug and food interactions.

Only very recently have pharmacologists and nutritionists become really interested in this special aspect of the relationship between drugs, food and nutrition. The first international congress on this subject was held only in 1976 [4]. Since 1981, a new journal devoted to this subject has been published [5].

Present Concepts of Food and Drug Relations

Food and drug relations might, a priori, be only conceived as a direct relationship restricted to the reciprocal actions of drugs and food in the alimentary canal. Actually, this view on the subject would be too narrow since many studies have shown that these relations implied all the phases of the drug and food metabolism as well as their alterations in relation to various nutritional states. On the other hand, for drugs interfering directly with the metabolism of drugs or their indirect effects on the system such as hypoglycemic substances, there exists a close chronology between the administration of the drug and the ingestion of food as well as a precise harmonization of the dosage with the amount and nature of the nutriments absorbed (carbohydrates in the present illustrative example). The effect of drugs is likely to vary according to the hormonal and metabolic state, and the dose administered is likely to differ between undernourished subjects and those under satisfactory nutritional conditions. It is also to be expected that dosage in obese subjects differ from that prescribed in individuals with normal body weight values, in particular for lipophilic or liposoluble drugs. It is not impossible that a severe body weight loss might release a number of these compounds, as shown for insecticides [6].

Particular attention should therefore be paid to the fate of drugs and food in the system at all stages so as to understand the nature and intensity of the relations between these two types of substances. It is therefore believed that if the possibility of administering drugs by an extradigestive route had partly brought about this disinterest for food and its effects, it was actually the wrong attitude, as shown by studies on the pharmacokinetics and metabolism of drugs.

These studies, however, are not easily conducted for various reasons which will be reviewed below. Man eats according to his own rhythm, usually 3, 4 or 5 times per day, sometimes only once or twice.

It is evident that the effects to be observed will depend not only on the temporal mode of alimentation but also on the specific chronopharmacology of the drug tested. The consequences of food intake on a family of drugs cannot be deduced from a study bearing only on one member of this family.

In view of severe interindividual variations, comparative studies are exploitable only if the subjects are their own controls. In addition, exposure to food and to the drug studied ought to be sufficiently long. It is well known in experimental nutrition that all studies carried out after a short change in dietary habits have no significant value as the system needs some time before its enzyme function and its hormone physiology adjust to the new nutritional conditions, as is the case with the administration of any drug.

These studies are expected to avoid changes in metabolic behavior under the influence of disease processes, otherwise the subjects could not be their own controls: such investigations must therefore be performed on healthy volunteers.

Such research is subject to considerable pressure: healthy volunteers are repeatedly exposed to the drug tested after nutritional preparation for approximately 3 weeks. Any aggressive drug is therefore banned, as is the case with research itself in a number of countries where studies on healthy human volunteers are prohibited.

For all these reasons, the works published are generally on single-dose studies conducted on subjects whose dietary regimens were modified from day to day. The interpretation of these studies is worth prudence.

Drug and Food Relations

A few examples reviewed below at very different stages of food and drug metabolism illustrate both the relevance of the subject matter and the precariousness of our knowledge in this field.

The Alimentary Canal as a Meeting Point

Drugs and food may interact either by increasing or decreasing absorption, or by altering their intradigestive metabolism. If such interactions are minor at the level of the mouth or the throat, they are more pronounced during intragastric passage. The amount of water, the temperature of food, the osmotic power of the meal, the nature of food (more particularly lipids), and the acidity or basicity of food alter the dissolution conditions of drugs and the rate of gastric emptying. Similarly, drugs may slow down the gastric emptying of food.

Food and drugs reach the intestine after a more or less lengthy interval and, according to their nature, will, if it is a question of lipids, or will not stimulate bile secretion. Due to their surface-active potential, bile salts will enhance the dissolution of some drugs in the gut and further the formation of a micellar medium favorable to the absorption of liposoluble drugs. This explains that bioavailability is increased when these drugs are taken during a fatty meal.

The intestine is evidently the preferential site of food and drug interactions. Food and drugs may chelate, neutralize, form insoluble complexes and precipitates. Antacids and covering agents intervene via their neutralizing power at all stages of dissolution, transformation and absorption of some drugs. The influence of food on the absorption of drugs is actually highly complex as it depends on the nature of the nutriments in food and on the mode of digestive absorption of drugs. If food influences drug absorption, it is the same with drugs on the absorption of food. There exist, however, drugs which demonstrate a major influence.

Drug-related changes in the digestive flora and their consequences upon food absorption have been studied in animals, but insufficiently in man to be able to draw clear conclusions [7]. These studies are all the more difficult as they are conducted on ill subjects and when infection is present the intradigestive metabolism of drugs may also be modified. The alimentary canal is therefore a direct meeting point for food and drugs. The nature and the intensity of the interactions depend on the nature of food and drugs but also on the rate of the passage into the different segments of the alimentary canal as they regulate the duration of contact of the substances in relation to one another and with the surface of the intestinal villosities.

The Presystemic Metabolism of Nutriments and Drugs

Nutriments (or simple elements in the composition of food) and drugs or their metabolites are carried in the portal venous blood to the liver. Most of them are transformed into metabolites under the influence of enzymes mostly present in the endoplasmic reticulum of the liver cells. The reactions of oxidation, reduction and conjugation constitute processes of detoxification to which esterases and the enzymatic systems of transmethylation of the liver microsomes contribute.

The activity of these liver enzyme systems varies according to genetic potential, sex, age and physiological conditions, and according to nutritional conditions, e.g. mode of alimentation, environmental substances of pollution, in particular xenobiotics ingested with food [8].

Many studies have shown to which extent variations in nutritional conditions could induce or repress the digestive, hepatic or pancreatic enzyme activities. The half-life of theophylline and antipyrine is reduced with a protein-enriched diet as compared with that observed with an isoenergetic diet rich either in carbohydrates or fats [9]. A diet supplemented with proteins or alcohol is known to increase the activity of the microsomal cytochrome P-450 system, while a carbohydrate-enriched diet induces an effect which is the very opposite.

In addition, drugs and food taken simultaneously increase blood flow in the liver. Thus, the pharmacological substances which are rapidly metabolized by the liver stop in it for a lesser time which increases their bioavailability.

Is There a Drug and Nutriment Competition at the Level of Plasma Binding?

Many drugs are carried in the blood after they have been bound to proteins. Actually, only small water-soluble molecules circulate freely. Among these proteins, plasma albumin plays a major role, alpha- and beta-lipoproteins a lesser one. A number of binding sites are known at present which are specific of various drug components of nutritional metabolites, fatty acids, amino acids, and metals. The modulation of the drug activity depends on the stability of the albumin binding since it makes it inactive. In undernourished subjects, hypoalbuminemia reduces the binding capacity of drugs [10]. Various nutriments, metabolites or hormone substances, the concentrations of which may vary according to the nutritional conditions, might a priori compete with the drugs.

They are bonded to specific proteins and do not interfere with albumin. On the other hand, a number of amino acids and non-esterified fatty acids, the concentrations of which are directly related to the nutritional state, bind to albumin. They might therefore compete with drugs ionized in blood which have the same binding sites by opposing their binding or by shifting them.

Can Food and Drug Interactions Be Noxious?

Food and drug interactions induce a decrease or an increase in digestive absorption, the activity of detoxification processes, or in the binding capacity to plasma albumin. They cause changes in the digestive absorption of drugs.

Besides these effects which involve consequences on drug bioavailability or the nutritional state, interactions exist which induce severe incidents or accidents: for instance, hypertensive attacks are often fatal, which results from interactions between monoamine oxidase inhibitors and food containing tyramine, or flush caused by alcohol taken concomitantly with hypoglycemic sulfonamides [11, 12], and the potentiation by alcohol of the hypnotic effects of sedatives: carcinogenic substances may form in the system from food nitrites originating in fertilizers which, by combining with the amine substances in food or drugs, form nitrosamines which are known to have a potent carcinogenic potential [13].

Mother's milk constitutes a poorly selective vector of drugs absorbed by the mother. Due to its metabolic immaturity, the effects of drugs on the system of the newborn may differ from those observed in adults.

Has the Nutritional State Any Influence on Drug Activity?

Under protein-energetic malnutrition conditions, there exist pharmacokinetic alterations secondary to changes in the liver and kidney metabolic functions and to the decrease in the binding capacity of drugs due to hypoalbuminemia [14, 15].

Intestinal absorption is also reduced for some nutriments such as carbohydrates [16] or drugs such as tetracycline. Clearance of antipyrine [17] is decreased under denutrition conditions, as is the case with the metabolism of antipyrine, isoniazide [18, 19], chloramphenicol [20] and digoxin [21].

The effects of denutrition on the metabolism of drugs seem to be different in children and adults. In the present state of knowledge, the results of these studies cannot yet be profitably used to modify the mode of drug prescription. The problems of obesity have not been solved because of insufficient supporting data. If obesity does not modify the conditions of digestive absorption, it likely involves an increase in the volumes of distribution, in particular when the drug is lipophilic, as already shown for antipyrine or diazepam [22, 23]. A fast of 15 days induces a decrease in the volume of distribution of drugs [24, 25]. Not enough investigations have been performed to clearly establish whether the metabolism of drugs is modified.

Conclusions

The relations between food, drugs and nutritional states are complex and still insufficiently known although they are of great importance. The occurrence of serious events gives sufficient cause for further studies in this new field.

The food and drug relations and their interactions may alter the therapeutic effects or the toxicity of drugs. They may also generate nutritional deficiencies in long-term treatments, more particularly in senescent subjects [26].

It is therefore necessary for pharmacologists and nutritionists to devote part of their research activities to this field. First of all, food and drugs, the interactions of which are both major and significant for practical therapeutic applications, have to be differentiated.

References

1 Vesell, E.S.; Shively, C.A.; Passananti, G.T.: The antipyrine test in clinical pharmacology: conceptions and misconceptions. Clin. Pharmacol. Ther. *26:* 275–286 (1979).
2 Vesell, E.S.; Page, J.G.: Genetic control of dicomarol levels in man. J. clin. Invest. *47:* 2657–2663 (1968).
3 Vesell, E.S.: Pharmacogenetics: multiple interactions between genes and environment as determinants of drug response. Am. J. Med. *66:* 183–187 (1979).
4 Nutrition and drug interrelations: The Nutrition Foundation (monograph series); in Hathcock, Coon, pp. 1–927 (Academic Press, New York 1978).
5 Drug and nutrient interactions (Liss, New York 1981).
6 Beaufrand, M.J.; Poullain, B.; Klein, D.; Debry, G.: Libération des pesticides organochlorés lors de pertes pondérales aigues. Tox. Eur. Res. *1:* 39–43 (1978).
7 Prins, R.A.: Nutritional impact of intestinal drug-microinteractions; in Hathcock, Coon, Nutrient and drug interrelations, pp. 319–345 (Academic Press, New York 1978).
8 Carr, C.J.: Food and drug interactions. Annu. Rev. Pharmacol. Toxicol. *22:* 19–29 (1982).
9 Anderson, K.E.; Conney, A.H.; Kappas, A.: Nutritional influences on chemical biotransformations in humans. Nutr. Rev. *40:* 161–171 (1982).

10 Shastri, A.R.; Krishnaswamy, K.: Undernutrition and tetracycline half-life. Clinica chim. Acta *66:* 157–164 (1976).
11 Royer, P.; Debry, G.; Lamarche, M.; Kissel, P.: Sulfamides hypoglycémiants et effets antabuse. Presse méd. *72:* 661–665 (1964).
12 Royer, R.; Debry, G.; Lamarche, M.: Recherches expérimentales sur les réactions vaso-motrices à l'alcool après administration de quelques sulfamides hypoglycémiants. Thérapie *17:* 989–997 (1962).
13 Klein, D.; Gaconnet, N.; Beaufrand, M.J.; Debry, G.: Formation des nitrosamines dans le tractus digestif humain. Evolution du pH et des concentrations en nitrates et nitrites dans le suc gastrique au cours de la digestion. Annls Nutr. Aliment. *30:* 813–821 (1976).
14 Buchanan, N.: Drug protein binding and protein energy malnutrition. S. Afr. med. J. *52:* 633–637 (1978).
15 Buchanan, N.: Drug kinetics in protein energy malnutrition. S. Afr. med. J. *53:* 327–330 (1978).
16 Gray, G.M.: Drugs, malnutrition and carbohydrate absorption. Am. J. clin. Nutr. *26:* 121–124 (1973).
17 Narang, R.K.; Metha, S.; Mathur, V.S.: Pharmacokinetic study of antipyrine in malnourished children. Am. J. clin. Nutr. *30:* 1979–1982 (1977).
18 Buchanan, N.; Eyberg, C.; Davis, M.D.: Isoniazid pharmacokinetics in kwashiorkor. S. Afr. med. J. *56:* 299–300 (1979).
19 Buchanan, N.; Davis, M.D.; Henderson, D.B.; Mucklow, J.C.; Rawlins, M.D.: Acetanilide pharmacokinetics in kwashiorkor. Br. J. clin. Pharmacol. *9:* 525–526 (1980).
20 Mehta, S.; Kalsi, H.K.; Jayaraman, S.; Mathur, V.S.: Chloramphenicol metabolism in children with protein-caloric malnutrition. Am. J. clin. Nutr. *28:* 977–981 (1975).
21 Buchanan, N.; Ven der Walt, L.A.; Strickwold, B.: Pharmacology of malnutrition. III. Binding of digoxin to normal and kwashiorkor serum. J. pharm. Sci. *65:* 914–916 (1976).
22 Abernethy, D.R.; Greenblatt, D.J.; Divoll, M.; Harmatz, J.S.; Shader, R.I.: Alterations in drug distribution and clearance due to obesity. J. Pharmac. exp. Ther. *217:* 681–685 (1981).
23 Abernethy, D.R.; Greenblatt, D.J.: Pharmacokinetics of drugs in obesity. Clin. Pharmacokinet. *7:* 108–124 (1982).
24 Reidenberg, M.J.M.; Kostenbauder, H.; Adams, W.P.: Rate of drug metabolism in obese volunteers before and during starvation and in azotemic patients. Metabolism *18:* 209–213 (1969).
25 Reidenberg, M.M.: Obesity and fasting-effects on drug metabolism and drug action in man. Clin. Pharmacol. Ther. *22:* 729–734 (1977).
26 Roe, D.A.: Dietary control of human studies related to aging and drug disposition or response. J. Am. Coll. Nutr. *1:* 199–205 (1982).

G. Debry, MD, Département de Nutrition et des Maladies Métaboliques de l'Université de Nancy I et Groupe Inserm U-59, 40, rue Lionnois, F–54000 Nancy (France)

Wld Rev. Nutr. Diet., vol. 43, pp. 10–33 (Karger, Basel 1984)

Food and Drug Interactions on Digestive Absorption

Peter Berchtold[a, b], *Thomas R. Weihrauch*[b], *Michael Berger*[a]

Department of Medicine E, [a]University of Düsseldorf;
[b]Department of Clinical Research, Bayer AG, Wuppertal, FRG

The intestinal tract is a major organ system responsible for the uptake, digestion and absorption of nutrients. Most drugs are given to the organism by the intestinal tract and therefore a high concentration of the drug may be available locally in the gut and interactions between intestinal cells and drugs occur. This review concentrates on interactions of drugs with food digestion and absorption and will consider the following: bile acid sequestering resins; dietary fiber; sucrose polyester; drugs that tend to cause malabsorption; drugs that cause maldigestion.

Bile Acid Sequestering Resins

Cholestyramine and colestipol are widely used for the treatment of hypercholesterolemia. About 15 g/day of colestipol appears to be equivalent to 12 g/day cholestyramine [56]. Both resins are not absorbed from the gut and exert their action by exchanging chloride ions for bile acids in the intestinal tract. The fecal excretion of bile acids markedly increases in normals [48] and in subjects with type II hyperlipoproteinemia [76]; the enterohepatic circulation of bile acids is interrupted. The main lipoprotein fractions affected are the low density lipoproteins (LDL) [73, 99]. High density lipoprotein (HDL)-cholesterol was not affected by cholestyramine (16 g/day); however, the plasma HDL_2/HDL_3 ratio and apolipoprotein AI concentration rose significantly, suggesting a beneficial effect to the recipient [99]. Fecal triglyceride content has been shown to be unchanged with 15-g/day doses, but with 30 g of cholestyramine administration up to 20 g or more fat may appear in the stool [47].

Dietary Fiber

At the moment there is great interest in dietary fiber and its effect on various metabolic and gastrointestinal parameters. This modern interest in fiber originates from the work of *Cleave* [24] who proposed that modern diseases were related to the intake of refined carbohydrates. *Burkitt* [16] found an association between increased colon cancer and decreased fiber intake and *Trowell* [105] correlated coronary heart disease with a decreased fiber intake. *Burkitt* [16] listed 8 conditions with high prevalence in the USA, but virtually non-existent in Africa: appendicitis, colon cancer, diverticular disease, gallstones, hemorrhoids, hiatus hernia, varicose veins and coronary heart disease. The difference in the occurrence of these diseases was attributed to the low intake of dietary fiber in the USA. Dietary fiber consists of plant cell materials which are not digested in the human upper gastrointestinal tract. Chemically they are non-carbohydrate lignin or polysaccharides, i.e. cellulose, hemicellulose, pectins, gums, mucilages or algal polysaccharides. Fibers hold water and when purified they can form gel in water, e.g. pectin, guar gum, certain hemicelluloses and mucilages (soluble fiber). Natural fiber products, such as vegetables, salads, fruits and bran, also hold water but do not usually form gel [75] (insoluble fiber, cellulose, lignins, certain hemicelluloses). For classification of fibers see table I. Different kinds of fiber regimens are under investigation for various indications:

Table I. Classification of fiber [adapted from ref. 67]

Class	Chemical components of main chain	
Cellulose	linear glucose polymer	carbohydrate
Hemicellulose	xylose, mannose, glucose, galactose	carbohydrate
Pectin[1]	galacturonic acid	carbohydrate
Gums[1]	galacturonic acid – rhamnose or mannose	carbohydrate
Mucilages[1]	galactose – mannose	carbohydrate
	galacturonic acid – rhamnose	carbohydrate
	arabinose – xylose	carbohydrate
Algal polysaccharides	mannose, xylose, glucose, glucuronic acid	carbohydrate
Lignin	sinapyl, coniferyl, coumaryl alcohols	non-carbohydrate

[1] Soluble.

Lipid Metabolism

The soluble fibers pectin and guar gum lower serum cholesterol levels in man, whereas cellulose and bran have no effect [66]. One possible mechanism of the hypolipemic action of fiber involves the binding of bile acids, which would result in reduced absorption of cholesterol, resulting in lower levels of cholesterol. Different types of fiber show variable effects in binding bile acids and bile salts [101]. A high binding capacity seems to correspond with a hypocholesteremic effect [100]. The effects of plant fibers on serum lipids in humans are described in table II [2].

Diabetes mellitus

Jenkins et al. [57, 58] clearly demonstrated that ingestion of carbohydrate with certain plant fibers result in a decrease of the postprandial glycemia in diabetics and normal volunteers. Guar was the most effective fiber, then, with decreasing effects, gum tragacanth and methylcellulose. The effects of pectin, bran and cholestyramine were negligible.

During glucose tolerance tests and following test meals the increase of postprandial serum insulin levels were less with fiber than without fiber. Long-term studies with high fiber diets (not soluble) in diabetics were performed by many groups [2] resulting in lower fasting, and postprandial blood glucose values, as well as lower insulin requirements. An increase in plant fiber intake can be readily achieved by substituting unrefined or min-

Table II. Effects of plant fibers on serum lipids in humans [1, 2]

Source of fiber	Number of studies	Plant fiber g/day	Fasting serum lipids % of control	
			cholesterol	triglycerides
Wheat bran	14	17	101	97
Bagasse	2	10.5	100	99
Cellulose	3	16	100	–
Whole oats	1	12	89	–
Psyllium	2	9.6	87	–
Pectin	10	25	87	99
Guar	3	24	84	–
Bengal gram	1	unknown	78	–
Multiple fibers	1	60	97	86
	1	unknown	84	76
	1	82	75	86

imally processed food for highly refined carbohydrates and fats. Long-term side effects on mineral and vitamin status have not been observed in one study [3]; however, more data are warranted. The long-term efficacy and safety of purified soluble fibers, such as guar and pectins, have not yet been demonstrated.

Colon Cancer

There is still controversy whether low levels of dietary fiber are associated with a high incidence of colonic cancer. Whereas *Burkitt* [17] favors this hypothesis, based on epidemiological evidence, *Drasar and Irving* [30] found no correlation between cancer of the colon and the breast and fiber intake.

It has been suggested that stool long delayed in its passage through the colon and rectum permits the development of carcinogens from normal dietary constituents by bacteria that may affect some normal constituents, such as bile salts, to produce lithocholic acid or some other noxious agent, which in turn could be responsible for cancer of the bowel [109]. There is evidence suggesting that a high intake of beef fat promotes the growth of intestinal bacteria, particularly bacterioides, which are more active at degrading cholesterol into carcinogens than are bacteria from the stool of persons on a low fat diet [32, 49]. Dihydroxycholanic acid is the metabolite considered to be at fault here. Deoxycholic and lithocholic acids are structurally related to certain carcinogens and clostridia are capable of producing carcinogens from bile acids [46]. *Hill* et al. [50, 51] could demonstrate a high bile acid concentration and fecal clostridia which can change those bile acids to carcinogens in over two thirds of patients with large bowel cancer, as contrasted with the same finding in less than 10% of patients with other diseases. Prospective studies documenting a decrease in the incidence of colon cancer through a fiber-rich diet are not yet available.

In summary, dietary fiber seems to exert a definitely beneficial effect in diabetes mellitus and some lipid disorders in man but a directly positive influence on cancer of the large bowel is still under discussion. The physiological actions of fiber are summarized in table III.

Sucrose Polyester

Sucrose polyester (SPE) is a fat like material consisting of a mixture of the hexa-, hepta- and octaesters formed by the reaction of sucrose with long chain fatty acids. This material is not hydrolyzed by the gastrointestinal enzymes and as a consequence it is not absorbed [39]. The material has the appearance and physical properties of the usual dietary fats. SPE was given in various dosages from 8 to 62 g/day. In normal volunteers a reduction of total and LDL-cholesterol of 10–19% was observed. A change in bile acid excretion or composition could not be demonstrated with SPE [40]. HDL-cholesterol and triglycerides were not changed with SPE. Vitamin A and E levels decreased by 10–21% [31, 39]. The effects of SPE in hypercholesterolemic subjects were not convincing [39]. A use of SPE as fat replacement in obese patients was suggested for weight reduction regimens [41].

Drugs that Tend to Cause Malabsorption

Biguanides

Biguanides have an effect on intestinal absorption processes. Biguanides are used in the treatment of maturity onset or type II diabetics [77] and/or hyperlipoproteinemia [44]. Effects of biguanides include a possible stimulation of glycogen deposition in the liver [13], inhibition of gluconeo-

Table III. Physiological actions of fiber [adapted from ref. 67]

Fiber class	Possible functions in man
Pectins, gums, and mucilages	slow gastric emptying, may bind bile acids, decrease serum cholesterol, improve glucose tolerance may affect trace mineral excretion
Hemicellulose	holds water; increases stool bulk may bind bile acids reduces elevated colonic intraluminal pressure reduces transit time
Cellulose	holds water may reduce colonic intraluminal pressure may affect trace mineral excretion reduces transit time
Lignin	possible antioxidant holds water may bind trace minerals affects fecal steroids

genesis [74], stimulation of glucose uptake in skeletal muscle [18] and inhibition of glucose absorption in the gut [28]. These effects can be explained by the work of *Schäfer* [95, 96] who showed that biguanides have a high affinity to mitochondrial membranes. Biguanides induce a retardation of cell respiration based on positive shift in membrane surface potentials. Recently a possible additional effect of biguanides was reported: the increase of the number of insulin receptors in different human cells [54, 81].

Intestinal Effects of Biguanides. The inhibition of glucose absorption was first demonstrated by *Czyzyk* et al. [28]. In mild type II diabetics glucose was administered orally and intravenously. In order to control slowed gastric emptying glucose was also given as an intraduodenal infusion. After oral and intraduodenal application phenformin induced a delay of the increase of postglucose glycemia, whereas after intravenous administration of glucose no change of the glucose disposal occurred. These results were confirmed by *Hollobaugh* et al. [55] and *Arvanitakis* et al. [4] in normal volunteers. *Caspary and Creutzfeldt* [20] demonstrated an inhibition of active sugar transport for all three biguanides: phenformin, buformin and metformin. We were interested whether other inhibitory effects could be observed in the intestinal tract. In patients with mild type II diabetes we found a significant decrease of the vitamin B_{12} absorption [8, 9, 62]. In addition, we found a moderate decrease of intestinal disaccharidase activities, namely of maltase, isomaltase and sucrase, which could also contribute to the intestinal effects of biguanides on carbohydrate absorption [9] (table IV). Effects of metformin indicating malabsorption of folic acid and ingested lipids were not as clearly demonstrated as the effects on vitamin B_{12} absorption. An impairment of vitamin B_{12} absorption during long-term treatment with phenformin and metformin was later confirmed by *Tomkin* [104] and *Tomkin* et al. [103] in diabetics. This impairment occurred in 30% of the patients treated with metformin and 46% of the patients treated with phenformin. *Willms and Creutzfeldt* [107] did not find vitamin B_{12} malabsorption during long-term treatment with buformin. Withdrawal of the biguanide treatment resulted in reversion of B_{12} absorption to normal in most patients examined [8, 103, 104]. Biguanides produced a prolongation of gastric emptying time in gastrectomized patients [46] with relief of dumping symptoms [45].

In our study on the intestinal effects of metformin [8] there was a tendency for higher fecal fat excretion during metformin treatment than before therapy. *Tomkin* et al. [103] described 1 patient with steatorrhea and a low

^{14}C-tripalmitate absorption test during metformin administration. When reexamined 4 weeks after withdrawal of metformin ^{14}C-tripalmitate absorption and fecal fat excretion had become normal. A recent study in rats demonstrated a reduction of the absorption of the fatty acid and glycerol moieties of ingested triglycerides by biguanides [27].

Cholchicine

Orally administered *cholchicine* produces widespread alterations of absorptive functions in humans as demonstrated by increased fecal loss of sodium, potassium, fat and nitrogen, by decreased absorption of *d*-xylose and vitamin B_{12} and by decreased serum cholesterol and carotene concentrations. Reduction of sucrase, maltase and lactase activity was found in mucosal tissue during cholchicine administration. All changes were reversible upon withdrawal of cholchicine [86].

Neomycin

This is another drug that induces malabsorption when given orally. Fat absorption is involved; some of this effect is also due to bile acid precipita-

Table IV. Schilling test and enzyme activities in intestinal biopsy specimens before (B) and after (A) Metformin treatment [9]

Patient	Age years	Time of treatment weeks		Schilling test %	Biopsy specimen enzyme activities in units/g protein (normal values in parentheses*)						
					maltase (266±70)	isomaltose (97±30)	sucrase (87±29)	trehalase	lactase (44±22)	acid β-galactosidase	hetero β-galactosidase
1	29	10	B	16.8	353	101	84	29	34	–**	–**
			A	0.8	140	46	36	15	18	3.9	3.0
2	47	2	B	15.3	355	133	99	34	39	4.2	<0.1
			A	5.5	135	52	35	15	19	4.1	1.0
3	25	5	B	19.0	183	81	50	24	34	4.1	2.2
			A	7.2	213	61	62	31	51	4.0	0.8
4	50	2	B	17.7	201	78	49	22	34	4.0	2.0
			A	5.5	213	82	57	25	52	4.3	2.8
5	52	2	B	19.2	269	84	67	35	53	5.3	4.9
			A	4.2	165	62	82	30	51	5.6	5.8
Mean			B	17.6	272	95	70	29	39	4.4***	2.3***
			A	4.6	173	61	54	23	38	4.5***	2.6***

* Mean ± SD (n = 22); ** not analyzed; *** patient 1 not included.

tion in the gut [106]. Vitamin B_{12} absorption and carbohydrate absorption are disturbed, the latter possibly due to lower disaccharidase activities [19, 34, 78].

Para-Aminosalicylic Acid

PAS was used in antituberculous therapy. A number of observers reported on its hypocholesterolemic effects [63, 68, 73, 94]. It became evident that PAS induced fat malabsorption although the PAS-induced steatorrhea did not correlate with its lipid lowering effect [71]. For the treatment of hyperlipoproteinemia a highly purified, in the presence of vitamin C recrystallized form, which was more palatable and had less gastrointestinal side effects [29] than older preparations, was used. Two groups achieved similar results in extensive studies with 8 g/day PAS-C® [7, 72] in the treatment of type IIa and type IIb hyperlipoproteinemia. A decrease was noted in total serum cholesterol, LDL-cholesterol and in serum triglycerides (table V) [7]. An additional effect of PAS in the gastrointestinal tract is an induction of vitamin B_{12} malabsorption [79, 80] without interfering with intrinsic factor.

The drugs which tend to cause malabsorption appear to induce mucosal changes [62]; however, there is no correlation between the degree of malabsorption or enzyme alteration and the degree of histologic change [86].

Table V. Serum lipid changes after long-term therapy with PAS-C® [7]

Duration of treatment	Cholesterol level mg/100 ml		Triglyceride level mg/100 ml	
	initial[1]	final	initial	final
6 months (n = 13)				
Mean ± SD	389 ± 116	319 ± 81	117 ± 46	85 ± 29
Change, mg/100 ml		−70		−32
p value		< 0.001		< 0.005
12 months (n = 7)				
Mean ± SD	406 ± 148	311 ± 98	121 ± 50	96 ± 20
Change, mg/100 ml		−95		−25
p value		< 0.005		n.s.

PAS-C = Para-aminosalicylic acid.

[1] Mean of three or four values during the 6 weeks preceding PAS-C value.

Drugs Inducing Maldigestion: Inhibitors of Intestinal α-Amylases and α-Glucosidases

The management of the so-called carbohydrate-dependent diseases, such as diabetes mellitus, obesity, and certain types of hypertriglyceridemia, is still far from satisfactory. In most diabetics postprandial blood glucose elevations are much higher than in normal subjects. A frequent problem in diabetics is the hyperglycemia in the morning hours after breakfast. It was hypothesized that a delay or inhibition of carbohydrate digestion in the intestinal tract and, therefore, decreased glucose absorption could be of use in diabetics in order to normalize or at least lower the postprandial blood glucose peaks more effectively. It is widely accepted today that improved metabolic control is important for diabetics in order to prevent large and especially small vessel disease [14, 37, 82]. Thus, any treatment with the attempt to normalize blood glucose levels should be evaluated. Since diabetics should avoid fast absorbable carbohydrates [25], like glucose and sucrose, the main carbohydrate in their diet should be starch, and a partial inhibition of starch digestion appeared to be appropriate.

α-Amylase Inhibitors

Mainly a non-protein amylase inhibitor was investigated: BAY e 4609 is a complex oligosaccharide of microbial origin [36, 84]. BAY e 4609 lowered in a dose-dependent way the postprandial glycemia and insulinemia in normal volunteers [84]. The highest dosage of 1.0 mega amylase inhibitor units (AIU) [36] led to an almost complete inhibition of glucose absorption. Also when standardized full meals with carbohydrate, protein and fat were served the amylase inhibitor decreased the postprandial blood glucose and insulin levels in normal volunteers in a dose-dependent manner. Similar results were reported for the circadian blood sugar profile in non-insulin-dependent diabetics [43]. In all of these studies there was a clear-cut effect of the amylase inhibitor BAY e 4609 on the postprandial glycemia and insulinemia in acute tests, using either starch or full meals without sucrose as a nutritional load. The effect of the inhibitor was reproducible after several meals during the day. Similar effects were obtained with trestatin, a new amylase inhibitor [65, 83] undergoing clinical testing.

In a pilot study on 3 insulin-dependent diabetics [*Willms,* 1975, unpublished results] no effect of the amylase inhibitor (3 × 0.6 mega AIU) was found on blood sugar or insulin dosage. Also in 16 obese non-insulin-dependent diabetics (NIDDM) 3 × 0.5 mega AIU used as a powder given together with the meals during 8 weeks did not produce clinically significant effects [*Frerichs, Jahnke,* 1975, unpublished results]. 6 patients complained of flatulence, 1 patient of meteorism. In other studies on diabetics, however, positive therapeutic effects could be demonstrated: in 10 NIDDM on sulfonylurea and/or biguanide treatment with poor control the addition of BAY e 4609 (0.6–1.2 mega AIU/meal) resulted in a significant ($p < 0.03$) decrease of the fasting and postprandial blood sugar and a reduction of the urine sugar after 8 weeks of treatment. Body weight and serum lipids did not change. 7 of the 10 patients reported soft stools [*Kaffarnik,* 1976, unpublished results].

In a study on patients with NIDDM not satisfactorily controlled with diet alone BAY e 4609 was administered as a powder together with meals (0.75–4.0 mega AIU/day) during 2 months (10 patients). 11 patients were treated with a placebo. Only postprandial blood glucose levels were significantly reduced whereas the fasting blood sugar and the blood sugar determined between 4 and 5 p.m. showed no changes [*Büber,* 1976, unpublished results]. In an uncontrolled pilot study on Japanese NIDDM BAY e 4609 1.5 mega AIU/day induced a decrease of the body weight and a marked reduction of the fasting and postprandial blood glucose [*Akazawa, Koide,* 1977, unpublished results]. The tolerability was excellent, no abdominal fullness, flatulence or diarrhea were reported. The very variable results observed in these studies reaching from no changes in the blood glucose profile to a marked lowering of the fasting and postprandial blood glucose and reduction of the body weight did not lead to the belief that an α-amylase inhibitor would be of substantial benefit to diabetic patients. The discrepancies in the different studies may be caused by different diets. In Japanese patients with a diet rich in starch and practically without refined sugars the best results were obtained, whereas in German patients considerable differences in the therapeutic efficacy were obtained. *Gries* et al. [42] tested diabetics on a diet with or free of mono- and disaccharides with and without BAY e 4609 and indeed found no effect of the inhibitor on blood glucose in patients on the mono- and disaccharide-containing diet. In contrast, patients on a mono- and disaccharide-free diet showed a marked reduction of the circadian glucose profile. It may be that the inhibitor showed no therapeutic efficacy because sucrose overcame its action on amylase digestion and sucrase was not inhibited by BAY e 4609. Another explanation could be a bad drug compliance. This was assessed by counting the tablets brought back by the patient at each investigation. Compliance was good and did not appear to be a reason for the failure of the drug.

Based on all these results it was decided to stop the further development of the α-amylase inhibitor BAY e 4609 because of inconsistent results and it was concluded that a sucrase inhibitor could be a more rational approach to so-called carbohydrate-dependent diseases than amylase inhibition alone [10].

The α-Glucosidase Inhibitor: Acarbose

In the laboratories of Bayer an α-glucosidase inhibitor, acarbose, was found [85]. A full report on all studies with acarbose was published recently [26]. Acarbose is a pseudo-tetrasaccharide prepared by fermentation from actinoplanacea. It inhibits the intestinal brush border enzymes sucrase, glucoamylase and maltase by competitive inhibition [22].

In many different clinico-pharmacological studies acarbose led to an inhibition or abolition of the postprandial increases of blood glucose, serum insulin and, in part, serum triglyceride levels [52, 102]. A mostly dose-dependent effect of acarbose was noted (fig. 1). In other studies it could be demonstrated that acarbose lowered not only serum insulin levels but also serum gastrointestinal polypeptide (GIP) [33, 35]. In addition it could be demonstrated in acute studies that acarbose effectively prolonged the absorption time of sucrose and that the amount of sucrose absorbed decreased [87]. In man acarbose decreased the absorption of sodium and water [23]. It was also noted that glucagon-like immunoreactivity (GLI) increased in a dose-dependent way with increasing acarbose dosage. This is probably related to the glucose stimulation of the gut hormone located in the intestinal tract by the maldigested sucrose or glucose [87]. Furthermore, acarbose increased breath hydrogen in normal volunteers, suggesting carbohydrate transfer into the colon and bacterial fermentation [21, 59, 60, 69, 70, 87].

In all clinico-pharmacological studies acarbose induced intestinal symptoms, such as flatulence, meteorism and in a limited amount of cases soft stools and diarrhea. In order to attenuate the symptoms, guar, dimethyl polysiloxane and an antacid, hydrotalcit, were tested with acarbose. No convincing results could be obtained [11].

An attempt to decrease colonic bacterial fermentation with neomycin resulted in a paradoxical increase of the intestinal symptoms, most probably due to a neomycin-induced malabsorption of sucrose and, secondly, because H_2 production may not predominantly be caused by a neomycin-sensitive organism and thirdly because neomycin may preferentially act on H_2-catabolizing bacteria and thus enhance hydrogen formation [34, 70]. Metronidazole significantly reduced acarbose-induced flatulence but not

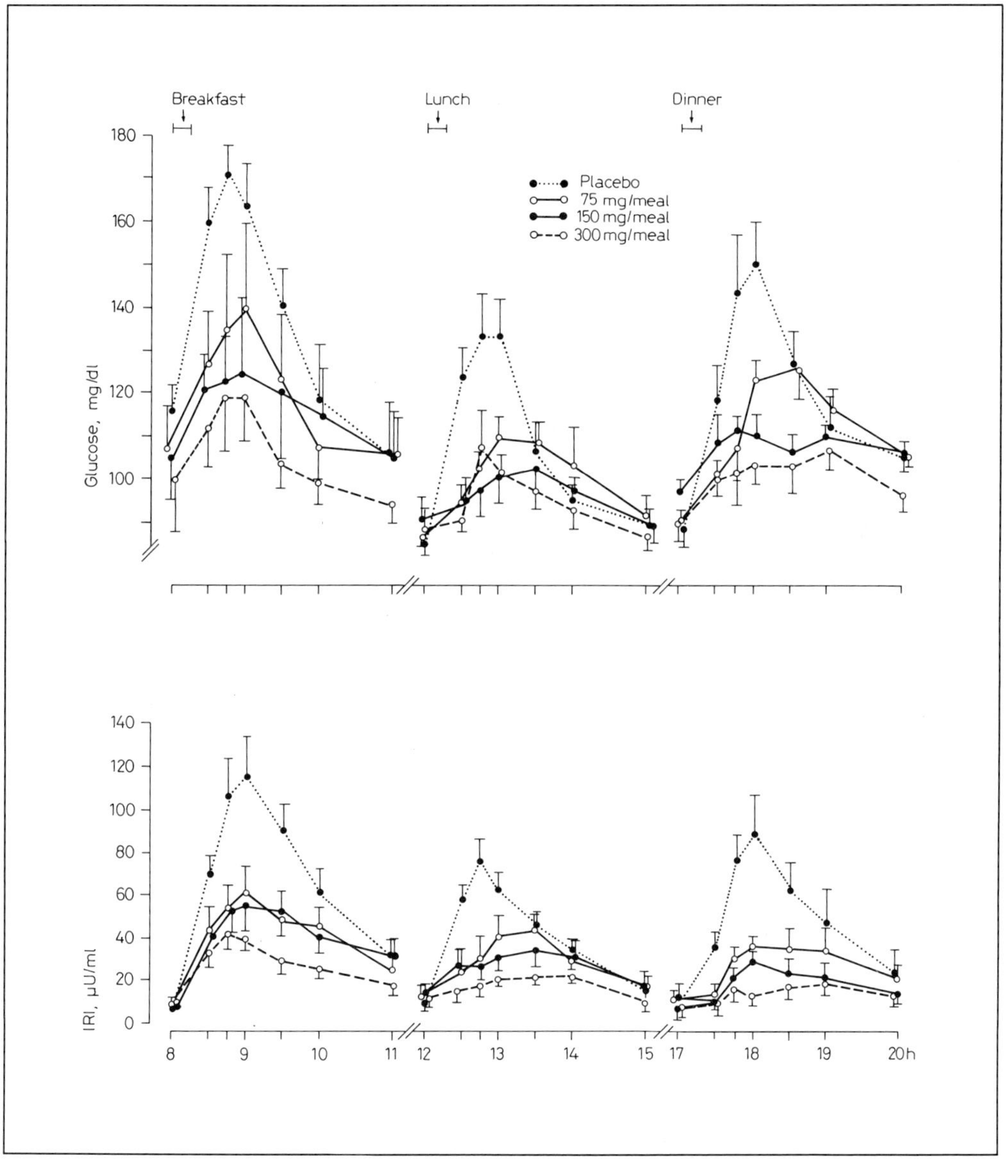

Fig. 1. Effects of acarbose on postprandial blood glucose and serum insulin levels in overweight volunteers during 3 mixed meals with 40% carbohydrates, 40% fat and 20% protein. Significant differences between the placebo and the acarbose treatment were found in all instances ($p < 0.05$) except for the glucose response to the 75 mg dosage after breakfast [12, 52].

meteorism and diarrhea [71]. Based on these results no drug can be recommended for the treatment of intestinal effects. Acarbose induces less intestinal symptoms and a later breath hydrogen evolution with pure starch loading tests than with sucrose loads [61, 103]; thus, it is advisable to decrease the sucrose- and increase the starch content of the diet when intestinal side effects become troublesome.

In clinical studies in both types of diabetes acarbose was shown to be effective in lowering postprandial blood glucose levels and, after a certain period, also fasting blood glucose levels [97]. Here we mention a few studies as examples of the effect of acarbose in diabetes.

Acarbose in Type I Diabetes. In a double-blind cross-over trial on patients with insulin-dependent diabetes mellitus (IDDM) acarbose was found to significantly reduce the diurnal blood sugar profile [90, 108] (fig. 2). Also other investigators found the blood glucose-lowering effect in IDDM: In 10 patients with IDDM without measurable C-peptide levels 200 mg acarbose per meal were administered up to 6 months. The efficacy of the drug was assessed by the artificial β-cell (Biostator). Before treatment, insulin requirements were 70 U/24 h compared with 38 after 1 month of

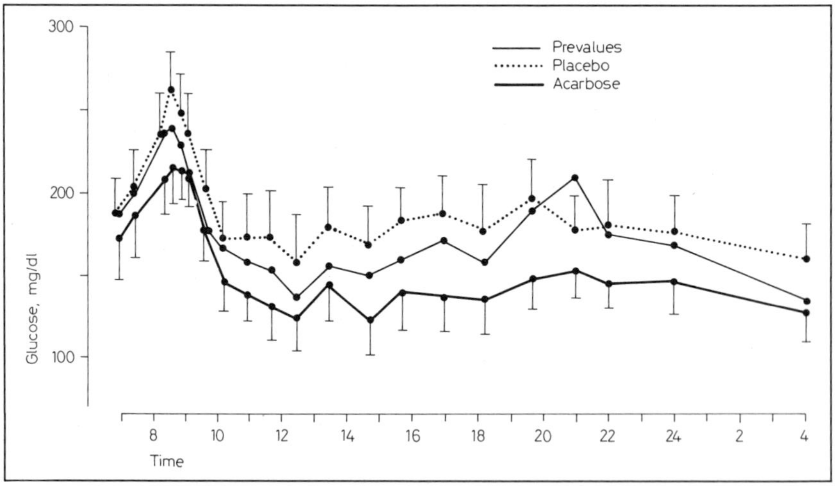

Fig. 2. Mean diurnal blood glucose values of 12 sulfonylurea-treated diabetics before treatment (thin solid line) and after 7 days' therapy with either acarbose (thick solid line) or placebo (dotted line). The bars represent 1 standard deviation. The integrated blood glucose response in mg/24 h was significantly decreased ($p < 0.05$) by acarbose [90].

treatment and 42 after 6 months of treatment. Blood sugar levels as well as serum triglyceride levels decreased substantially during treatment; in addition catecholamine and cortisol levels were reduced [88]. When 10 patients with IDDM were taken off additional biguanide treatment and developed poor control, acarbose was given and effectively decreased blood glucose levels. It was concluded that acarbose could replace biguanide treatment in these patients [98]. In 28 patients with IDDM acarbose was given over a 2-month period, preceded and followed by a 2-month placebo period. Acarbose significantly decreased the mean daily blood glucose, the mean amplitude of glucose excursion and the M-value. Acarbose reduced postbreakfast and postdinner blood glucose values by 25% ($p < 0.001$) and 24% ($p < 0.05$), respectively [38].

Acarbose in Type II Diabetes. In order to test whether different frequencies of drug application would induce different metabolic responses, 10 patients with NIDDM received either placebo or 100 mg of acarbose 3 times/day or 50 mg 6 times/day in an 8-day cross-over trial. Drug efficacy was examined by continuous blood glucose monitoring (glucogram). There was a significant decrease of glycemia during acarbose treatment, but there was no difference between the two drug application frequencies [92]. In another study, it was compared whether acarbose would be equally effective when given 200 mg once per day or 200 mg t.i.d. and it could be demonstrated that both regimens were equally effective, except that in the once-per-day group the blood glucose levels after dinner were not as well controlled as in patients receiving the drug with each meal [108]. Lowering effects of acarbose on different parameters of glucose metabolism were obtained in 12 sulfonylurea-treated patients (table VI) [90]. 20 patients with

Table VI. Fasting, mean and maximum blood glucose, integrated blood glucose response and amplitude of glycemic excursions in 12 orally treated diabetics (mean ± SEM). p-values for the comparison of acarbose to placebo are given (n.s. = not significant) [90]

	Initial values	Placebo	Acarbose	p
Fasting blood glucose, mg/dl	163 ± 18.8	141 ± 16.7	130 ± 18.2	n.s.
Mean blood glucose, mg/dl	231 ± 15.3	230 ± 12.1	192 ± 10.4	<0.001
Maximum blood glucose, mg/dl	162 ± 12.1	157 ± 12.4	140 ± 10.7	<0.005
Integrated blood glucose response, mg/dl × 21 h	3,564 ± 235	3,421 ± 201	3,112 ± 191	<0.005
Amplitude of glycemic excursions, mg/dl	123 ± 9.5	129 ± 6.1	96 ± 6.4	<0.005

Table VII. Effects of drugs and dietary fiber on nutrient assimilation in man

Drug	Principal biologic action, indication	Effect on carbohydrate assimilation
Cholestyramine Colestipol	cholesterol lowering agent, hypercholesterolemia	–
Dietary fiber Soluble: guar	diabetes type I and II, hypercholesterolemia	bind water and therewith glucose; improve glucose tolerance
Pectin	as guar but less effective	small, improving effect on glucose tolerance
Insoluble: cellulose, bran	bind water, influence intestinal transit time	–
Biguanides	diabetes type II, hyperlipoproteinemia	inhibition of glucose absorption, reduction of disaccharidase activity (?), *d*-xylose malabsorption
Cholchicine	antiinflammatory alcaloid for the treatment of gouty arthritis	reduction of disaccharidase activity, *d*-xylose malabsorption
Neomycin	antibiotic	reduction of disaccharidase activity, especially lactase
PAS	antitubercular drug	–
BAY d 7791 BAY e 4609 Trestatin	α-amylase inhibitors	inhibition of α-amylase improve starch tolerance
Acarbose	α-glucosidase inhibitor (diabetes type I and II) dumping syndrome, reactive hypoglycemia, hypertriglyceridemia	inhibition of sucrase, maltase, gluco-amylase, improve sucrose and starch tolerance by delayed intestinal absorption

Table VII. (cont.)

Effect on fat assimilation	Effect on vitamin absorption and others	Reference(s)
bile acid sequestering interruption of enterohepatic circulation, lower serum cholesterol	–	47, 48, 56, 76, 89
bind bile acid, lower serum cholesterol	–	57, 58, 66
bind bile acid, lower serum cholesterol	–	57, 58
–	–	57, 58, 66
inhibition of fat absorption, lower serum cholesterol and triglycerides	inhibition of B_{12} and (?), folic acid absorption	8, 9, 20, 27, 28, 103, 104, 107
inhibition of fat absorption lower serum cholesterol and carotene	B_{12} malabsorption Na, K, N malabsorption	86
bile acid precipitation decrease fat absorption	B_{12} malabsorption	19, 34, 78, 106
fat malabsorption, lower serum cholesterol and triglycerides	B_{12} malabsorption	7, 71, 72, 79, 80
some decrease of serum triglycerides (?)	–	64, 65, 83, 84
lower serum triglycerides	sodium and water absorption inhibited	11, 12, 22, 26, 85, 87

NIDDM, treated with diet alone or with sulfonylurea compounds, were assigned to a double-blind cross-over trial with 8-week periods. Acarbose (0.4–1.0 g/day) and placebo treatment were compared. An oral 75-gram sucrose load was used to assess drug efficacy, and blood glucose and serum insulin levels were determined. Blood glucose levels were significantly decreased [15] and a significant improvement of the sucrose tolerance was observed although on the test day the patients did not receive acarbose. Serum insulin levels during the sucrose tolerance test were increased in 10 patients. This, however, did not reach statistical significance in the whole group. Nevertheless, this points to the possibility that with continuous acarbose therapy there may be an improved function of the β-cell in some of the patients. In a study of 6 NIDDM patients, a substantial fall in the circadian blood glucose profile could be obtained [93]. It is of note that in this study no change in serum insulin levels was observed.

In a long-term study 12 patients on sulfonylurea were additionally treated with acarbose [93]. After a 3-month preperiod a 6-month treatment period was followed by another 3-month period without acarbose. There was a marked decrease of the postprandial blood sugar. The fasting blood sugar remained unaffected. HbA_1 was significantly decreased during the treatment period.

In most studies, intestinal side effects became apparent, but disappeared with prolonged treatment time [91]. 60–70% of all patients show some intestinal effects of the drug. With continuous treatment time, however, the symptoms are decreasing. No adverse side effects regarding clinical biochemistry or hematology have been observed up to now [53].

From a long-term study, which was performed by 16 general practitioners on 245 patients, results of 143 patients were collected, in whom all blood glucose values were available. There was a marked drop of fasting and postprandial blood glucose levels. After 1 year of treatment a placebo phase was added and the blood glucose values reincreased again [6]. Also in this study it was shown that side effects decreased with prolonged treatment time. Only 5% of the patients dropped out because of intolerable intestinal side effects. Biochemical and hematological values remained unchanged [5].

Not all diabetics, however, responded favorably to acarbose. Up to a quarter to a third of the patients were, for yet unknown reasons, 'non-responders'.

Table VII displays an overview of the drugs presented in this chapter.

References

1 Anderson, J.W.; Chen, W.L.: Plant fiber. Carbohydrate and lipid metabolism. Am. J. clin. Nutr. *32:* 346–363 (1979).

2 Anderson, J.W.; Midgley, W.R.; Wedman, B.: Fiber and diabetes. Diabetes Care *2:* 369–379 (1979).

3 Anderson, J.W.; Ferguson, S.K.; Karonnos, D.; O'Malley, L.; Sieling, B.; Chen, W.L.: Mineral and vitamin status on high-fiber diets: long-term studies of diabetic patients. Diabetes Care *3:* 38–40 (1980).

4 Arvanitakis, C.; Lorenzsonn, V.; Olsen, W.A.: Phenformin-induced intestinal function and mitochondrial structure in man. J. Lab. clin. Med. *82:* 195–200 (1973).

5 Aubell, R.; Boehme, K.; Berchtold, P.: Blood glucose concentration and glycosuria during and after one year of acarbose therapy. Drug Res. *33:* 1314–1318 (1983).

6 Aubell, R.; Boehme, K.; Berchtold, P.: One-year acarbose treatment of diabetic outpatients. Multicenter study part II: efficacy; in Creutzfeldt, 1st Int. Symp. on Acarbose, pp. 363–366 (Excerpta Medica, Amsterdam 1982).

7 Barter, P.J.; Connor, W.E.; Spector, A.A.; Armstrong, M.; Connor, S.A.; Newman, M.A.: Lowering of serum cholesterol and triglyceride by para-aminosalicylic acid in hyperlipoproteinemia. Ann. intern. Med. *81:* 619–624 (1974).

8 Berchtold, P.; Bolli, P.; Arbenz, U.; Keiser, G.: Intestinale Absorptionsstörung infolge Metforminbehandlung. Diabetologia *5:* 405–412 (1969).

9 Berchtold, P.; Dahlquist, A.; Gustafson, A.; Asp, N.-G.: Effects of a biguanide (metformin) on vitamin B_{12} and folic acid absorption and intestinal enzyme activities. Scand. J. Gastroent. *6:* 751–754 (1971).

10 Berchtold, P.; Kiesselbach, N.H.K.: The clinical significance of the alpha-amylase inhibitors BAY d 7791 and BAY e 4609; in Berchtold, Cairella, Jacobelli, Silano, Regulators of intestinal absorption in obesity, diabetes and nutrition, pp. 181–200 (Soc. Editrice Universo, Roma 1981).

11 Berchtold, P.; Hillebrand, I.; Boehme, K.; Aubell, R.; Nagel, L.; Schulz, H.: The clinical significance of the α-glucosidase inhibitor acarbose; in Berchtold, Cairella, Jacobelli, Silano, Regulators of intestinal absorption in obesity, diabetes and nutrition, pp. 261–280 (Soc. Editrice Universo, Roma 1981).

12 Berchtold, P.; Hillebrand, I.: Clinical pharmacology of an α-glucosidase inhibitor: acarbose; in Melish, Hanna, Baba, Genetic and environmental interaction in diabetes mellitus, pp. 332–335 (Excerpta Medica, Amsterdam 1982).

13 Beringer, A.; Geyer, G.; Mösslacher, H.; Tragl, K.H.; Thaler, H.: Die Wirkung von Buformin auf den Leberstoffwechsel; in Oberdisse, Daweke, Michael, 2. Int. Biguanid-Symp., pp. 43–49 (Thieme, Stuttgart 1968).

14 Brownlee, M.; Cahill, G.F.: Diabetic control and vascular complication. Atheroscler. Rev. *4:* 29–70 (1979).

15 Büber, V.: Effect of acarbose in non-insulin-dependent diabetic patients during long-term treatment; in Creutzfeldt, 1st Int. Symp. on Acarbose, pp. 266–274 (Excerpta Medica, Amsterdam 1982).

16 Burkitt, D.P.: Related diseases – related cause. Lancet *ii:* 1229–1231 (1969).

17 Burkitt, D.P.: Colonic-rectal cancer: fiber and other dietary factors. Am. J. clin. Nutr. *31:* 58–64 (1978).

18 Butterfield, W.J.; Wichelow, M.J.: The hypoglycemic action of phenformin. Diabetes *11:* 281–286 (1962).
19 Cain, G.D.; Reiner, E.B.; Patterson, M.: Effects of neomycin on disaccharidase activity of the small bowel. Archs intern. Med. *122:* 311–319 (1968).
20 Caspary, W.F.; Creutzfeldt, W.: Analysis of the inhibitory effect of biguanides on glucose absorption: inhibition of active sugar transport. Diabetologia *7:* 379–385 (1971).
21 Caspary, W.F.: Sucrose malabsorption in man after ingestion of α-glucoside-hydrolase inhibitor. Lancet *i:* 1231–1233 (1978).
22 Caspary, W.F.; Graf, W.: Inhibition of human intestinal α-glucosidehydrolases by a new complex oligosaccharide. Res. exp. Med. *175:* 1–6 (1979).
23 Caspary, W.F.; Kalisch, H.: Effect of α-glucosidase inhibition on intestinal absorption of sucrose, water and sodium in man. Gut *20:* 750–755 (1979).
24 Cleave, T.L.: The neglect of natural principles in current medical practice. J. R. naval med. Serv. *42:* 55–82 (1956).
25 Crapo, P.A.; Reaven, G.A.; Olefsky, J.: Plasma glucose and insulin responses in orally administered simple and complex carbohydrates. Diabetes *25:* 741–747 (1976).
26 Creutzfeldt, W.: Proceedings of the First International Symposium on Acarbose. Excerpta Med. Int. Congr. Ser., No. 594 (1982).
27 Curtis-Prior, P.B.: Reduction of the absorption of the fatty acid and glycerol moieties of ingested triglycerides by biguanides. Int. J. Obesity *6:* 299–306 (1982).
28 Czyzyk, A.; Tawecki, J.; Sadowski, J.; Ponikowska, J.; Szczepanik, Z.: Effects of biguanides on intestinal absorption of glucose. Diabetes *17:* 492–498 (1968).
29 Donnerberg, R.L.; Browning, R.H.; Atwell, R.J.: Studies of conjugated PAS ascorbic acid and other forms of para-aminosalicylic acid. I. Patient tolerance. Am. Rev. Tuberc. pulm. Dis. *76:* 877–879 (1957).
30 Drasar, B.S.; Irving, D.: Environmental factors and cancer of the colon and breast. Br. J. Cancer *27:* 167–172 (1973).
31 Fallat, R.W.; Glueck, C.J.; Luttmer, R.; Mattson, F.H.: Short-term study of sucrose polyester, a non-absorbable fat-like material as a dietary agent for lowering plasma cholesterol. Am. J. clin. Nutr. *29:* 1204–1215 (1976).
32 Finegold, S.M.; Sutter, V.L.; Sugihara, P.T.; Elder, H.A.; Lehmann, S.M.; Philips, R.L.: Fecal microbial flora in Seventh Day Adventist populations and control subjects. Am. J. clin. Nutr. *30:* 1781–1792 (1977).
33 Fölsch, U.R.; Ebert, R.; Creutzfeldt, W.: Response of serum levels of gastric inhibitory polypeptide and insulin to sucrose ingestion during long-term application of acarbose. Scand. J. Gastroent. *16:* 629–632 (1981).
34 Fölsch, U.R.; Lembcke, B.; Caspary, W.F.; Ebert, R.; Creutzfeldt, W.: Influence of neomycin on postprandial metabolic changes of a glucoside-α-hydrolase inhibitor (Acarbose); in Berchtold, Cairella, Jacobelli, Silano, Regulators of intestinal absorption in obesity, diabetes and nutrition, vol. 2, pp. 249–258 (Soc. Editrice Universo, Roma 1981).
35 Fölsch, U.R.; Lembcke, B.; Ebert, R.; Caspary, W.F.; Creutzfeldt, W.: Effects of acarbose and fibre on glucose and hormone response to sucrose load or mixed meal; in Creutzfeldt, 1st Int. Symp. on Acarbose, pp. 96–106 (Excerpta Medica, Amsterdam 1982).

36 Frommer, W.; Puls, W.; Schaefer, D.; Schmidt, D.: DOS 206 4092 (1972).
37 Fuller, H.; Shipley, M.J.; Rose, G.; Jarret, R.J.; Keen, H.: Coronary heart disease risk and impaired glucose tolerance. Lancet *i:* 1373–1376 (1980).
38 Gérard, J.; Luyckx, A.S.; Lefèbvre, P.J.: Improvement of metabolic control in insulin-dependent diabetics treated with the α-glucosidase inhibitor acarbose for two months. Diabetologia *21:* 446–451 (1981).
39 Glueck, C.J.; Mattson, F.H.; Jandacek, R.J.: The lowering of plasma cholesterol by sucrose polyester in subjects consuming diets with 800, 300 or less than 50 mg of cholesterol per day. Am. J. clin. Nutr. *32:* 1636–1644 (1979).
40 Glueck, C.J.; Jandacek, R.J.; Subbiah, M.T.R.; Gallon, L.; Yunker, R.; Allen, C.; Hogg, E.; Laskarzewski, P.M.: Effect of sucrose polyester on fecal bile acid excretion and composition in normal men. Am. J. clin. Nutr. *33:* 2177–2181 (1980).
41 Glueck, C.J.; Hastings, M.M.; Allen, C.; Hogg, E.; Baehler, L.; Gartside, P.S.; Phillips, D.; Jones, M.; Hollenbach, E.J.; Braun, A.S.; Anastasia, J.V.: Sucrose polyester and covert caloric dilution. Am. J. clin. Nutr. *35:* 1352–1359 (1982).
42 Gries, F.A.; Grüneklee, D.; Drost, H.: On the effects of glucosidase inhibitors in diabetes mellitus. Front. Horm. Res., vol. 7, pp. 265–275 (Karger, Basel 1980).
43 Grüneklee, D.; Elze, W.; Gries, F.A.: Wirkung eines α-Amylaseinhibitors auf Blutglukosetagesprofile bei manifestem Diabetes und standardisierter Ernährung; in Jahnke, Mehnert, Metabolische und klinische Aspekte der Kohlenhydrate in der Ernährung, pp. 92–95 (Kirchheim, Mainz 1973).
44 Gustafson, A.; Björntorp, P.; Fahlen, M.: Metformin administration in hyperlipidemic states. Acta med. scand. *190:* 491–496 (1971).
45 Gyr, K.; Berger, W.; Göschke, H.; Stalder, G.: Postprandiale Beschwerden nach Gastrektomie und ihre Beeinflussung durch Dimethylbiguanid. Dt. med. Wschr. *48:* 2421–2431 (1970).
46 Gyr, N.; Berger, W.; Fridrich, R.; Denes, A.; Stalder, G.A.: Der Einfluss von Dimethylbiguanid auf die Magenentleerung und die orale Glukosetoleranz. Schweiz. med. Wschr. *101:* 1876–1879 (1971).
47 Hashim, S.A.; Bergen, S.S.; VanItallie, T.B.: Experimental steatorrhea induced in man by bile acid sequestrants. Proc. Soc. exp. Biol. Med. *106:* 173–175 (1961).
48 Hashim, S.A.; VanItallie, T.B.: Cholestyramine resin therapy for hypercholesterinemia. J. Am. med. Ass. *192:* 289–293 (1965).
49 Hill, M.J.: Colon cancer – a disease of fiber depletion and dietary excess. Digestion *11:* 298–306 (1975).
50 Hill, M.J.; Drasar, B.; Aires, V.; Crowther, J.; Hawksworth, G.; Williams, R.: Bacteria and aetiology of cancer of the large bowel. Lancet *i:* 95–100 (1975).
51 Hill, J.M.; Drasar, B.S.; Williams, R.; Meade, T.W.; Cox, A.G.; Simpson, J.E.; Morson, B.C.: Faecal bile acids and colistrida in patients with cancer of the large bowel. Lancet *i:* 535–538 (1975).
52 Hillebrand, I.; Boehme, K.; Frank, G.; Fink, H.; Berchtold, P.: The effects of the α-glucosidase inhibitor BAY g 5421 (Acarbose) on meal-stimulated elevation of circulating glucose, insulin and triglyceride levels in man. Res. exp. Med. *175:* 81–86 (1979).
53 Hillebrand, I.; Boehme, K.: Clinical studies on acarbose during 5 years; in Creutzfeldt, 1st Int. Symp. on Acarbose, pp. 445–450 (Excerpta Medica, Amsterdam 1982).

54 Holle, A.; Mangels, W.; Dreyer, M.; Kühnau, J.; Rüdiger, H.W.: Biguanide treatment increases the number of insulin receptor sites on human erythrocytes. New Engl. J. Med. *305:* 563–566 (1981).
55 Hollobaugh, S.L.; Rao, M.B.; Kruger, F.A.: Studies on the site and mechanism of action of phenformin. Diabetes *19:* 45–49 (1970).
56 Hunninghake, D.B.; Probstfield, J.L.: Drug treatment of hyperlipoproteinemia; in Rifkind, Levy, Hyperlipoproteinemia, diagnosis and therapy, pp. 327–382 (Grune & Stratton, New York 1977).
57 Jenkins, D.J.A.; Leeds, A.R.; Gassull, M.A.; Wolever, T.M.S.; Goff, D.V.; Alberti, K.G.M.M.; Hockaday, T.D.R.: Unabsorbable carbohydrates and diabetes: decreased postprandial hyperglycemia. Lancet *ii:* 172–174 (1976).
58 Jenkins, D.J.A.; Leeds, A.R.; Gassull, M.A.; Cochet, B.; Alberti, K.G.M.M.: Decrease in postprandial insulin and glucose concentrations by guar and pectin. Ann. intern. Med. *86:* 20–23 (1977).
59 Jenkins, D.A.; Taylor, R.H.; Nineham, R.; Goff, D.V.; Bloom, S.R.; Sarson, D.; Alberti, K.G.M.M.: Combined use of guar and acarbose in reduction of postprandial glycemia. Lancet *ii:* 924–927 (1979).
60 Jenkins, D.J.A.; Taylor, R.H.; Goff, D.V.; Fielden, H.; Misiewicz, J.J.; Sarson, D.L.; Bloom, S.R.; Alberti, K.G.M.M.: Scope and specificity of acarbose in slowing carbohydrate absorption in man. Diabetes *30:* 951–954 (1981).
61 Jenkins, D.J.A.; Taylor, R.H.: Acarbose: dosage and interaction with sugars, starch and fibre; in Creutzfeldt, 1st Int. Symp. on Acarbose, pp. 86–96 (Excerpta Medica, Amsterdam 1982).
62 Keiser, G.; Berchtold, P.; Bolli, P.; Arbenz, U.: Störung der Vitamin-B_{12}-Absorption infolge Biguanidtherapie. Schweiz. med. Wschr. *100:* 351–353 (1970).
63 Kerstill, J.; Svanborg, A.: Treatment of hypercholesterolemia with para-aminosalicylic acid. Acta med. scand. *186:* 539–544 (1966).
64 Kiesselbach, N.H.K.; Puls, W.; Keup, U.: Effect of a new α-amylase inhibitor (BAY e 4609) on postprandial glycemia and insulinemia in non-diabetic male volunteers eating standardized meals. Diabetologia *10:* 372 (1974).
65 Korn, A.; Eichler, H.G.; Gasic, S.; Pirson, W.; Businger, J.: Effect of Trestatin (Ro 09-0154) a new alpha-amylase inhibitor on postprandial blood glucose and insulin levels in man. Diabetologia *23:* 181 (1982).
66 Kritchevsky, D.: Fiber, lipids and atherosclerosis. Am. J. clin. Nutr. *31:* 65–74 (1978).
67 Kritchevsky, D.: Dietary fiber and disease. Bull. N.Y. Acad. Med. *58:* 230–241 (1982).
68 Kuo, P.T.; Fan, W.C.; Kostis, J.B.; Hayase, K.: Combined para-aminosalicylic acid and dietary therapy in long-term controls of hypercholesterolemia and hypertriglyceridemia (types IIa and IIb hyperlipoproteinemia). Circulation *53:* 338–341 (1976).
69 Lembcke, B.; Caspary, W.R.; Hönig, M.; Frerichs, H.; Ebert, R.; Creutzfeldt, W.: Effect of carbohydrate gelling agents in addition to an α-glucosidehydrolase inhibitor on postprandial blood glucose, IRI, GIP, and intestinal H_2 production. Front. Horm. Res., vol. 7, pp. 293–294 (Karger, Basel 1980).
70 Lembcke, B.; Caspary, W.R.; Fölsch, U.R.; Creutzfeldt, W.: Influence of neomycin on postprandial metabolic changes and side effects of an α-glucosidehydrolase inhib-

itor (BAY g 5421). I. Effects on intestinal hydrogen gas production and flatulence. Front. Horm. Res., vol. 7, pp. 294–295 (Karger, Basel 1980).
71 Lembcke, B.; Fölsch, U.R.; Caspary, W.F.; Creutzfeldt, W.: Influence of metronidazole on intestinal side effects of acarbose; in Creutzfeldt, 1st Int. Symp. on Acarbose, pp. 236–238 (1982).
72 Levine, R.A.: Steatorrhea induced by para-aminosalicylic acid. Ann. intern. Med. *68:* 1265–1270 (1968).
73 Levy, R.I.; Langer, T.: Hypolipidemic drugs and lipoprotein metabolism. Adv. exp. Med. Biol. *26:* 155–163 (1972).
74 Meyer, F.; Ipaktchi, H.; Clauser, A.: Specific inhibition of gluconeogenesis by biguanides. Nature, Lond. *213:* 203–204 (1967).
75 Miettinen, T.A.: Effects of dietary fiber on serum lipids and cholesterol metabolism in man; in Gotto, Smith, Allen, Atherosclerosis V, pp. 311–315 (Springer, Berlin 1980).
76 Moore, R.B.; Crane, C.A.; Frantz, I.D.: Effect of cholestyramine on the fecal excretion of intravenously administered cholesterol-4-^{14}C and its degradation products in a hypercholesterolemic patient. J. clin. Invest. *47:* 1664–1671 (1968).
77 Oberdisse, K.; Daweke, H.; Michael, G.: 2. Int. Biguanid-Symp. (Thieme, Stuttgart 1968).
78 Paes, I.C.; Searl, P.; Rubert, M.W.; Faloon, W.W.: Intestinal lactase deficiency and saccharide malabsorption during oral neomycin administration. Gastroenterology *53:* 49–58 (1967).
79 Palva, I.P.; Heinivaara, O.; Mattila, M.: Drug-induced malabsorption of vitamin B_{12}. Scand. J. Haemat. *3:* 149–153 (1966).
80 Palva, I.P.; Rytkönen, U.; Alatulkkila, M.; Palva, H.L.A.: Drug-induced malabsorption of vitamin B_{12}. Scand. J. Haemat. *9:* 5–7 (1972).
81 Pezzino, V.; Trischitta, V.; Purello, F.; Vigneri, R.: Effect of metformin on insulin binding to receptors in cultured human lymphocytes and cancer cells. Diabetologia *23:* 131–135 (1982).
82 Pickup, J.C.; Keen, H.: The value of good control. Ir. J. med. Sci. *148:* suppl. 2, pp. 54–62 (1979).
83 Pirson, W.; Buschschacher, P.: Pharmacological properties of trestatin, a new α-amylase inhibitor. Diabetologia *21:* 315 (1981).
84 Puls, W.; Keup, U.: Metabolic studies with an amylase inhibitor in acute starch loading tests in rats and men and its influence on the amylase content of the pancreas; in Howard, Recent advances in obesity research, vol. I, pp. 391–393 (Newman, London 1975).
85 Puls, W.; Keup, U.; Krause, H.P.; Müller, L.; Schmidt, D.D.; Thomas, G.; Truscheit, E.: Pharmacology of a glucosidase inhibitor. Front. Horm. Res., vol. 7, pp. 235–247 (Karger, Basel 1980).
86 Race, T.F.; Paes, I.C.; Faloon, W.W.: Intestinal malabsorption by oral cholchicine. Am. J. med. Sci. *259:* 32–41 (1970).
87 Radziuk, J.; Kemmer, F.; Berchtold, P.; Vranic, M.: Quantitation of the effects of the α-glucosidase inhibitor acarbose on the hydrolysis and absorption of sucrose and hormone responses in man; in Creutzfeldt, 1st Int. Symp. on Acarbose, pp. 113–122 (Excerpta Medica, Amsterdam 1982).
88 Raptis, S.; Dimitriadis, G.; Karaiskos, C.; Diamantopoulos, E.; Hadjidakis, D.; Sou-

vatzoglou, A.; Moulopoulos, S.: Short- and long-term studies of acarbose on various metabolic parameters and insulin requirements assessed by the artificial endocrine pancreas; in Creutzfeldt, 1st Int. Symp. on Acarbose, pp. 393–401 (Excerpta Medica, Amsterdam 1982).

89 Ryan, J.R.; Jain, A.K.; McMahon, F.G.: Long-term treatment of hypercholesterolemia with colestipol hydrochloride. Clin. Pharmacol. Ther. *17:* 83–87 (1975).

90 Sachse, G.; Willms, B.: Effect of the α-glucosidase inhibitor BAY g 5421 on blood glucose control of sulfonylurea-treated diabetics and insulin-treated diabetics. Diabetologia *17:* 287–290 (1979).

91 Sachse, G.; Mäser, E.; Laube, H.; Federlin, K.: Effect of long-term acarbose therapy on the metabolic situation of sulphonylurea-treated people; in Creutzfeldt, 1st Int. Symp. on Acarbose, pp. 298–304 (Excerpta Medica, Amsterdam 1982).

92 Sailer, D.; Röder, G.: Treatment of non-insulin-dependent diabetic adults with a new glycoside hydrolase inhibitor (BAY g 5421). Drug Res. *30:* 1282–1285 (1980).

93 Sailer, D.: The influence of a new glucoside hydrolase inhibitor on blood glucose and serum insulin concentration in non-insulin treated diabetics. Hormone metabol. Res. *13:* 57 (1981).

94 Samuel, P.; Waithe, W.I.: Reduction of serum cholesterol concentration by neomycin, para-aminosalicylic acid, and other antibacterial drugs in man. Circulation *24:* 578–582 (1961).

95 Schäfer, G.: On the mechanism of action of hypoglycemia-producing biguanides: a re-evaluation and a molecular theory. Biochem. Pharmacol. *25:* 2005–2014 (1976).

96 Schäfer, G.: Some new aspects of the interactions of hypoglycemia producing biguanides with biological membranes. Biochem. Pharmacol. *25:* 2015–2024 (1976).

97 Schöffling, K.; Hillebrand, I.; Berchtold, P.: Treatment of diabetes mellitus with the glycoside hydrolase inhibitor acarbose (BAY g 5421). Front. Horm. Res., vol. 7, pp. 248–257 (Karger, Basel 1980).

98 Schwedes, U.; Petzoldt, R.; Haupt, E.; Hillebrand, I.; Schöffling, K.: Metabolic effect of acarbose in poorly controlled insulin-dependent diabetic out-patients after withdrawal of biguanides; in Creutzfeldt, 1st Int. Symp. on Acarbose, pp. 494–499 (Excerpta Medica, Amsterdam 1982).

99 Shepherd, J.; Packard, C.J.; Morgan, H.G.; Third, J.L.H.C.; Stewart, J.M.; Lawrie, T.D.V.: The effects of cholestyramine on high density lipoprotein metabolism. Atherosclerosis *33:* 433–444 (1979).

100 Story, J.A.; Kritchevsky, D.: Comparison of the binding of various bile acids and bile salts in vitro by several types of fiber. J. Nutr. *106:* 1292–1294 (1976).

101 Story, J.A.; Kritchevsky, D.: Bile acid metabolism and fiber. Am. J. clin. Nutr. *31:* 199–202 (1978).

102 Taylor, R.H.; Jenkins, D.J.A.; Barkett, H.M.; Fielden, H.; Goff, D.V.; Misiewicz, J.J.; Lee, D.A.; Allen, H.B.; MacDonald, G.; Wallrabe, H.: Effect of acarbose on the 24-hour blood glucose profile and pattern of carbohydrate absorption. Diabetes Care *5:* 92–96 (1982).

103 Tomkin, G.H.; Hadden, D.R.; Weaver, J.A.; Montgomery, D.A.D.: Vitamin B_{12} status of patients on long-term metformin therapy. Br. med. J. *ii:* 685–687 (1971).

104 Tomkin, G.H.: Malabsorption of vitamin B_{12} in diabetic patients treated with phenformin: a comparison with metformin. Br. med. J. *iii:* 673–675 (1973).

105 Trowell, H.: Coronary heart disease and dietary fiber. Am. J. clin. Nutr. *28:* 798–799 (1975).
106 Truswell, A.S.: Drugs and lipid metabolism. Proc. Nutr. Soc. *33:* 215–224 (1974).
107 Willms, B.; Creutzfeldt, W.: Contribution to the intestinal resorption of vitamin B_{12} (Schilling test) and of *d*-xylose in biguanide treatment. Diabetologia *6:* 652 (1970).
108 Willms, B.; Sachse, G.; Unger, H.: Treatment of diabetes with a glycoside hydrolase inhibitor (Acarbose, BAY g 5421). Front. Horm. Res., vol. 7, pp. 276–281 (Karger, Basel 1980).
109 Winder, E.L.; Reddy, B.S.: The epidemiology of cancer of the large bowel. Am. J. dig. Dis. *19:* 937–946 (1974).

Prof. P. Berchtold, Sandoz AG, CH–4002 Basel (Switzerland)

Wld Rev. Nutr. Diet., vol. 43, pp. 34–44 (Karger, Basel 1984)

Influence of Food and Different Nutrients on Drug Bioavailability[1]

A. Melander

Division of Clinical Pharmacology, Lund University Health Sciences Center, Dalby, Sweden

Drug Bioavailability

The bioavailability of a drug denotes how much of the administered dose that reaches systemic circulation, and hence can be distributed to the tissues for subsequent action. Usually, bioavailability signifies oral bioavailability, as oral intake is by far the most common route of drug administration.

For many drugs, bioavailability is incomplete and subject to inter- and intraindividual variation for reasons related both to the drug and its formulation and to the patient and his/her status and habits. After ingestion of tablets, these must disintegrate before the drug can be dissolved from the tablet particles. This dissolution has to occur either in the acid gastric juice or in the more alkaline environment of the small intestine before the drug can be absorbed, i.e. pass through the gastrointestinal wall into the portal circulation. It is generally assumed that most drugs are absorbed by passive diffusion through lipoprotein membranes; hence, the disintegration-dissolution-absorption processes are governed by the tablet formulation and by

[1] Most studies cited in this review have been supported by Grant No. 3880 from the Swedish Medical Research Council, and by grants from the Swedish Board of Health and Welfare and from the Swedish Delegation for Social Research (the Dalby project).

the acid-base character and pK_a of the drug in question. In addition, some drugs can also be absorbed by active transport mechanisms [15]. Causes for incomplete drug absorption can be sought among each of these facets.

Even though drug absorption per se may be complete, the bioavailability of a drug can be grossly impaired because it is metabolically transformed already during the first passage through the gastrointestinal mucosa and the liver. Such presystemic elimination occurs mainly with lipophilic basic drugs, such as antidepressants and some of the β-adrenergic antagonists [21], but also with esterified acids, such as acetylsalicylic acid [7]. In the case of propranolol, presystemic elimination may reduce bioavailability to 20–30%. In extreme cases, such as dihydroergotamine, there is both incomplete absorption and extensive presystemic metabolism, resulting in almost non-existent oral bioavailability [5].

Influence of Food on Drug Bioavailability

Food may influence both absorption and presystemic metabolism of drugs, and these effects may be caused by food intake as such, by different nutrients in the food, by additives and preservatives, by different fluids and fluid volumes, and by polycyclic hydrocarbons present in grilled or smoked food. The influence on absorption is usually related to changes in gastric emptying and/or gastrointestinal pH, in turn affecting tablet disintegration and drug dissolution. The influence on presystemic metabolism may relate to changes in splanchnic-hepatic blood flow but also to nutrients and additives in the diet. It should be emphasized in this context that 'food' may signify very different kinds of meals, and that one type of meal or food component may have both qualitatively and quantitatively different effects on drug bioavailability than another. Moreover, different formulations of the same drug may interact differently with food. From the clinical point of view, it is also urgent to emphasize that findings based on single-meal, single-dose studies in healthy volunteers need not yield relevant information as to effects of food on the steady-state concentrations and effects of a drug during long-term treatment in patients.

With the above-mentioned precautions in mind, this report will summarize the influence of a standardized breakfast meal on the bioavailability of a number of common drugs. Most of these data are derived from studies in our own laboratory, where healthy young volunteers (25–40 years old) have participated in bioavailability studies after fasting overnight (at least

Table I. Content of standardized breakfast used in most studies cited

Food	Content
150 ml low fat milk 100 ml orange juice 1 boiled egg 2 pieces of crisp rye bread 5 g saturated margarine 20 g orange marmalade 20 g hard cheese 100 ml non-sweetened black coffee or tea	= 20 g (20% protein, 17 g (35%) fat, 50 g (45%) carbohydrate = 1,840 kJ = 440 kcal

12 h) and following ingestion of a single oral dose of the drug in question both during continued fasting (2–4 additional hours) and together with a breakfast of 1,840 kJ (table I). Blood samples were obtained before and at numerous intervals after drug ingestion, and the plasma or serum concentrations of the drug were determined with selective, sensitive methods. Various kinetic parameters were calculated, in particular the area under concentration (AUC) curve, which is proportional to the amount of drug entering systemic circulation. Accordingly, an intraindividual AUC ratio (non-fasting/fasting) being significantly above or below 1.0 indicates a food-induced increase or decrease in drug bioavailability. In principle, studies in other laboratories have employed a similar approach.

Enhancement of Drug Absorption by Food

As shown in table II, several drugs have shown an increased bioavailability when ingested together with the standardized breakfast described. In some of these cases, it seems probable that the increased bioavailability is due to enhanced absorption. Among these drugs is phenytoin (as a micronized preparation of phenytoin acid), for which a 25% increase was recorded [22]. A more pronounced effect was seen with a non-micronized preparation of the anticoagulant dicoumarol; its bioavailability was enhanced by about 85% [20]. A slight increase has been reported for the diuretic hydrochlorothiazide [3], the urinary antiseptic nitrofurantoin [2, 35] and the antipsoriatic agent methoxypsoralen [10].

Table II. Influence of food intake on drug bioavailability

Drug	Effect of food	Probable cause
Dicoumarol	increased bioavailability	enhanced absorption
Hydrochlorothiazide	increased bioavailability	enhanced absorption
Methoxypsoralen	increased bioavailability	enhanced absorption
Nitrofurantoin	increased bioavailability	enhanced absorption
Phenytoin	increased bioavailability	enhanced absorption
Hydralazine	increased bioavailability	reduced presystemic metabolism
Labetalol	increased bioavailability	reduced presystemic metabolism
Metoprolol	increased bioavailability	reduced presystemic metabolism
Propranolol	increased bioavailability	reduced presystemic metabolism
Ampicillin	decreased bioavailability	reduced absorption
Atenolol	decreased bioavailability	reduced absorption
Isoniazid	decreased bioavailability	reduced absorption
Penicillin V	decreased bioavailability	reduced absorption
Rifampicin	decreased bioavailability	reduced absorption
Tetracyclines	decreased bioavailability	reduced absorption
Acetylsalicylic acid (aspirin)	decreased bioavailability	
Metronidazole	no change	
Nitrazepam	no change	
Oxazepam	no change	
Propylthiouracil	no change	
Salicylate[1]	no change	
Warfarin	no change	

[1] NB difference from aspirin!

All these drugs are more or less lipophilic compounds with incomplete absorption in the fasting state. Hence it seems likely that the enhanced bioavailability in the non-fasting state may result from a food-induced delay in gastric emptying, allowing for better dissolution of the drug [23]. Indeed, this notion is supported by studies indicating that anticholinergic pretreatment mimics the effect of food [4, 14]. In the case of phenytoin, special conditions may apply, as this drug is absorbed not only by passive diffusion but also via active transport [15], and as different nutrients may have opposite effects on phenytoin absorption (see below).

Reduction of Drug Absorption by Food

As shown in table II, the absorption of some drugs is impaired instead of enhanced by food intake. Among these agents are some chemotherapeutic agents, such as isoniazid [24], rifampicin [1], tetracyclines [31] and ampicillin [32, 41] – but not the ampicillin ester pivampicillin [34] – and one β-adrenoceptor blocker, atenolol [25]. At least for some of these drugs, the decreased bioavailability seems to be due to impaired dissolution subsequent to reduced gastric acidity; in support of this, it has been shown that antacid drugs have an effect similar to that of food intake [13, 33].

Acetylsalicylic acid (ASA) is an especially intriguing example of the complex interactions of food and drugs. ASA is a strong analgesic, antipyretic and anti-platelet agent, but its effect is markedly reduced when taken orally, because it is rapidly and extensively deacetylated to the much weaker agent salicylic acid (SA) already in the first passage through gut and liver [7]. The degree of this conversion varies greatly between rapid- and slow-release preparations of ASA, the former supplying much more unchanged ASA than the latter. In addition, food intake can markedly reduce the exposure to ASA, because of the delay in drug absorption [unpublished].

Drugs Unaffected by Food Intake

As shown in table II, there are also several drugs whose bioavailability seems to be unaffected by concomitant food intake. Among these are the anxiolytic/hypnotic agents nitrazepam [12] and oxazepam [26], the anticoagulant warfarin [unpublished data], the antimicrobials metronidazole [27] and sulfaisodimidine [23], and the antithyroid agent propylthiouracil [29].

Enhanced Drug Bioavailability Due to Reduced Presystemic Metabolism

Several drugs that are lipophilic bases undergo metabolism already in the first passage through gut and liver, and this presystemic clearance can drastically reduce their bioavailability. It has been demonstrated that concomitant food intake enhances the bioavailability of some drugs in this category, such as the β-adrenoceptor antagonists propranolol [21], metoprolol [21], and labetalol [9], and the vasodilator hydralazine [30]. On the other hand, food exerts little or no influence on the bioavailability of amitriptyline, codeine, *d*-propoxyphene, prazosin and zimelidine, even though these drugs, like the β-blockers, are lipophilic bases with pronounced presystemic clearance [28]. As the former are metabolized by hydroxylation, glucuronidation or acetylation but the latter by demethylation, it seems possible that concomitant intake of food (protein) may selectively inhibit acetylation, hydroxylation and glucuronidation without affecting demethylation. Indeed, the increase in propranolol bioavailability is proportional to the protein content of the food [40].

A contributing factor is the transient increase in splanchnic-hepatic blood flow that occurs following food intake [18, 28]. This may allow more unmetabolized drug to escape presystemic elimination [18, 28], and it is of interest in this context that hydralazine, which in itself increases splanchnic-hepatic blood flow, can enhance the bioavailability of propranolol [19]. Moreover, the apparent selectivity of the enzyme inhibition by food may in fact be secondary to an acute increase of the splanchnic-hepatic drug concentration, exceeding the saturation level of capacity-limited enzyme systems in the liver [28].

Influence of Different Nutrients on Drug Bioavailability

Rather few studies have addressed the question whether the influence of food relates to food intake as such or rather to some specific nutrient. One study has shown that a fat-rich meal enhances the absorption of griseofulvin, but that no such effect is seen with a low-fat diet [8]. The enhanced effect of food on phenytoin absorption seems related to the presence of carbohydrates, since intake of carbohydrate increases, while intake of protein reduces, phenytoin bioavailability [16]. Intake of fat had no measurable influence [16]. It is possible that this relates to the fact that phenytoin may be absorbed by an active transport mechanism, also employed by glucose [15].

Insofar as the influence of food on presystemic metabolism is concerned, there is evidence to suggest that the reduction of the presystemic elimination of propranolol is proportional to the amount of protein in the diet [40].

Influence of Food Additives, Preservatives and Contaminants on Drug Bioavailability

In addition to food and different nutrients, also additives, preservatives and, in particular, contaminants such as polycyclic hydrocarbons from grilling and smoking may alter drug bioavailability [*Alvares,* this volume].

Dissimilar Effects of Food on Drugs with Similar Actions

As previously described, food intake enhances the bioavailability of at least three β-adrenoceptor blockers, namely propranolol, metoprolol and labetalol. On the other hand, concomitant food intake reduces the bioavailability of another β-blocker, atenolol. This emphasizes that generalizations cannot automatically be made as to the effect of food intake on related drugs, at least not based upon similarity of action. Rather, the effect of food is determined by physicochemical properties of the drugs. In the case of β-blockers, food intake enhances the bioavailability of those agents that are completely absorbed but are subject to extensive presystemic metabolism. As food reduces presystemic metabolism, the concomitant food intake enhances the bioavailability of these three agents. Atenolol, on the other hand, escapes presystemic metabolism, but its absorption is incomplete already in the fasting state and becomes further impaired in combination with food.

Food may even have different effects on one and the same drug when given in different formulations; the bioavailability of salicylate was markedly reduced when taken together with food in a conventional enteric-coated formulation but was unaffected when the drug was administered in a slow-release preparation based on individually coated granules [6]. In addition, some erythromycin preparations have shown reduced bioavailability of this drug in connection with food intake [11], while food reportedly improves rather than impaires the absorption of erythromycin given as the stearate [17].

Clinical Significance of Food Influence on Drug Bioavailability

In most cases pharmacotherapy involves long-term oral administration of a drug in order to attain a steady-state level which should be within the therapeutic interval, i.e. sufficiently high to give the requested effect but sufficiently low to avoid untoward effects. During most circumstances, the rate of drug entry into systemic circulation has little or no clinical relevance; the relevant factors are the extent of bioavailability and the rate of drug elimination. Accordingly, the influence of food on drug bioavailability is clinically relevant only insofar as the alteration in drug bioavailability forces the steady-state level outside the therapeutic interval. Accordingly, it seems likely that the influence of food on drug bioavailability is clinically important only when the influence is very drastic, e.g. in the case of hydralazine, or when the therapeutic interval is very narrow, e.g. phenytoin and dicoumarol. It should also be emphasized that, although there is now a fair amount of data concerning the influence of food on single-dose bioavailability, there is almost no information as to the influence of food intake on the steady-state concentrations and therapeutic effects of drugs. Such studies are necessary to assess the clinical significance of the influence of food on drug bioavailability.

There are, on the other hand, certain drugs whose effects are dependent not only upon the extent of bioavailability but also on their rate of entry into systemic circulation. Among these agents are rapid-acting hypnotics and antidiabetic agents. In such cases, food intake may have an important influence on the clinical response to the drug. Thus, the sleep-inducing effect of pentobarbital is delayed by concomitant food intake [39]. On the other hand, food intake does not measurably effect the rate of entry of the two benzodiazepines, nitrazepam and oxazepam [12, 26]. The relations between food and antidiabetic sulfonylureas are discussed in the next section.

Influence of Food Intake on the Bioavailability and Effect of Sulfonylureas

In the treatment of diabetes mellitus, adequate relations between the intake of food and that of drugs should be essential, because food intake and the composition of the ingested food plays a major role in the control of this disease. Recent studies show that food intake has little or no influence on the extent of bioavailability of the sulfonylureas tolbutamide, chlorpropamide, glibenclamide and glipizide [36, 37, 42]. However, the rate of glipizide absorption is markedly delayed by concomitant food intake, and administration of glipizide half an hour before breakfast promotes a better blood glucose control due to more appropriate timing of insulin release than does intake of the drug together with the meal [42]. Moreover, even though the absorption rate of glibenclamide seems unaffected by food, also the effect of this drug is improved by administration half an hour before breakfast [38].

Conclusions

(1) Concomitant intake of food may alter both the rate of drug entry and the extent of drug bioavailability.

(2) This influence may be exerted both on the absorption and on the presystemic metabolism of drugs, and it may be subsequent to food intake as such or to different nutrients.

(3) Food intake can have different effects on drugs having similar actions but different physicochemical properties. Different effects may also occur with one and the same drug if given in different formulations.

(4) Even though food intake may markedly alter drug bioavailability in single-dose studies, this need not signify that this difference has clinical relevance in the sense that the steady-state concentrations and drug effects are compromised. Therefore, it should be mandatory to assess the influence of food intake on the bioavailability of each new drug and each new formulation; moreover, if such an effect is recorded in single-dose studies, the influence of food should also be assessed with respect to steady-state concentrations and therapeutic effects of the drug.

References

1 Acocella, G.: Clinical pharmacokinetics of rifampicin. Clin. Pharmacokinet. *3:* 128–143 (1978).

2 Bates, T.R.; Sequeira, J.A.; Tembo, A.V.: Effect of food on nitrofurantoin absorption. Clin. Pharmacol. Ther. *16:* 63–68 (1974).

3 Beermann, B.; Groschinsky-Grind, M.: Gastrointestinal absorption of hydrochlorothiazide enhanced by concomitant intake of food. Eur. J. clin. Pharmacol. *13:* 125–128 (1978).

4 Beermann, B.; Groschinsky-Grind, M.: Enhancement of the gastrointestinal absorption of hydrochlorothiazide by propantheline. Eur. J. clin. Pharmacol. *13:* 385–387 (1978).

5 Bobik, A.; Jennings, G.; Skews, H.; Esler, M.; McLean, A.: Low oral bioavailability of dihydroergotamine and first-pass extraction in patients with orthostatic hypotension. Clin. Pharmacol. Ther. *30:* 673–679 (1981).

6 Bogentoft, C.; Carlsson, I.; Ekenved, G.; Magnusson, A.: Influence of food on the absorption of acetylsalicylic acid from enteric-coated dosage forms. Eur. J. clin. Pharmacol. *14:* 351–355 (1978).

7 Brantmark, B.; Wåhlin-Boll, E.; Melander, A.: Bioavailability of acetylsalicylic acid and salicylic acid from rapid- and slow-release formulations, and in combination with dipyridamol. Eur. J. clin. Pharmacol. *22:* 309–314 (1982).
8 Crounse, R.G.: Effective use of griseofulvin. Archs Derm. *87:* 176–180 (1963).
9 Daneshmend, T.K.; Roberts, C.J.C.: The influence of food on the oral and intravenous pharmacokinetics of a high clearance drug: a study with labetalol. Br. J. clin. Pharmacol. *14:* 73–78 (1982).
10 Ehrsson, H.; Nilsson, S.-O.; Ehrnebo, M.; Wallin, I.; Wennersten, G.: Effect of food on kinetics of 8-methoxypsoralen. Clin. Pharmacol. Ther. *25:* 167–171 (1979).
11 Hirsch, H.H.; Finland, M.: Effect of food on the absorption of erythromycin propionate, erythromycin stearate and triacetyloleandomycin. Am. J. med. Sci. *237:* 693–699 (1959).
12 Holm, V.; Melander, A.; Wåhlin-Boll, E.: Influence of food and of age on nitrazepam kinetics. Drug Nutr. Interact. *1:* 307–311 (1982).
13 Hurwitz, A.: Antacid therapy and drug kinetics. Clin. Pharmacokinet. *2:* 269–280 (1977).
14 Jaffe, J.M.: Effect of propantheline on nitrofurantoin absorption. J. pharm. Sci. *64:* 1729–1730 (1975).
15 Johansson, Ö.; Lindberg, T.; Melander, A.: In vivo absorption of phenytoin from rat small intestine and its inhibition by phlorizin. Acta pharmac. tox. *45:* 265–271 (1979).
16 Johansson, Ö.; Wåhlin-Boll, E.; Lindberg, T.; Melander, A.: Opposite effects of carbohydrate and protein on phenytoin absorption in man. Drug Nutr. Interact. *2:* 139–144 (1983).
17 Malmborg, A.-S.: Absorption of erythromycin stearate after oral administration. Curr. med. Res. Opin. *5:* suppl. 2, pp. 15–18 (1978).
18 McLean, A.J.; McNamara, P.J.; duSouich, P.; Gibaldi, M.; Lalka, D.: Food, splanchnic blood flow, and bioavailability of drugs subject to first-pass metabolism. Clin. Pharmacol. Ther. *24:* 5–10 (1978).
19 McLean, A.; Skews, H.; Bobik, A.; Dudley, F.J.: Interaction between oral propranolol and hydralazine. Clin. Pharmacol. Ther. *27:* 726–732 (1980).
20 Melander, A.; Wåhlin, E.: Enhancement of dicoumarol bioavailability by concomitant food intake. Eur. J. clin. Pharmacol. *14:* 441–444 (1978).
21 Melander, A.; Danielson, K.; Schersten, B.; Thulin, T.; Wåhlin, E.: Enhancement of the bioavailability of propranolol and metoprolol by food. Clin. Pharmacol. Ther. *22:* 108–112 (1977).
22 Melander, A.; Brante, G.; Johansson, Ö.; Lindberg, T.; Wåhlin-Boll, E.: Influence of food on the absorption of phenytoin in man. Eur. J. clin. Pharmacol. *15:* 269–274 (1969).
23 Melander, A.: Influence of food on the bioavailability of drugs. Clin. Pharmacokinet. *3:* 337–351 (1978).
24 Melander, A.; Danielson, K.; Hanson, A.; Jansson, L.; Rerup, C.; Scherstén, B.; Thulin, T.; Wåhlin, E.: Reduction of isoniazid bioavailability in normal men by concomitant intake of food. Acta med. scand. *200:* 93–97 (1976).
25 Melander, A.; Stenberg, P.; Liedholm, H.; Scherstén, B.; Wåhlin-Boll, E.: Food-induced reduction in bioavailability of atenolol. Eur. J. clin. Pharmacol. *16:* 327–330 (1979).

26 Melander, A.; Danielson, K.; Vessman, J.; Wåhlin, E.: Bioavailability of oxazepam: absence of influence of food intake. Acta pharmac. tox. *40:* 584–588 (1977).

27 Melander, A.; Kahlmeter, G.; Kamme, C.; Ursing, B.: Bioavailability of metronidazole in fasting and non-fasting healthy subjects and in patients with Crohn's disease. Eur. J. clin. Pharmacol. *12:* 69–72 (1977).

28 Melander, A.; McLean, A.J.: Influence of food intake on presystemic clearance of drugs. Clin. Pharmacokinet. *8:* 286–297 (1983).

29 Melander, A.; Wåhlin, E.; Danielson, K.; Hanson, A.: Bioavailability of propylthiouracil: interindividual variation and influence of food intake. Acta med. scand. *201:* 41–44 (1977).

30 Melander, A.; Danielson, K.; Hanson, A.; Rudell, B.; Scherstén, B.; Thulin, T.; Wåhlin, E.: Enhancement of hydralazine bioavailability by food. Clin. Pharmacol. Ther. *22:* 104–107 (1977).

31 Neuvonen, P.J.: Interactions with the absorption of tetracyclines. Drugs *11:* 45–54 (1976).

32 Pierpaoli, P.G.: Drug therapy and diet. Drug Intell. clin. Pharm. *6:* 89–99 (1972).

33 Regårdh, C.G.; Lundborg, P.; Persson, B.-A.: The effect of antacid, metoclopramide and propantheline on the bioavailability of metoprolol and atenolol. Biopharm. Drug Disp. *2:* 79–87 (1981).

34 Roholt, K.; Nielsen, B.; Kristensen, E.: Clinical pharmacology of pivampicillin. Antimicrob. Agents Chemother. *6:* 563–571 (1974).

35 Rosenberg, H.A.; Bates, T.R.: The influence of food on nitrofurantoin bioavailability. Clin. Pharmacol. Ther. *20:* 227–232 (1976).

36 Sartor, G.; Melander, A.; Scherstén, B.; Wåhlin-Boll, E.: Influence of food and age on the single-dose kinetics and effects of tolbutamide and chlorpropamide. Eur. J. clin. Pharmacol. *17:* 285–293 (1980).

37 Sartor, G.; Melander, A.; Scherstén, B.; Wåhlin-Boll, E.: Serum glibenclamide in diabetic patients, and influence of food on the kinetics and effects of glibenclamide. Diabetologia *18:* 17–22 (1980).

38 Sartor, G.; Lundquist, I.; Melander, A.; Scherstén, B.; Wåhlin-Boll, E.: Improved effect of glibenclamide on administration before breakfast. Eur. J. clin. Pharmacol. *21:* 403–408 (1982).

39 Smith, R.B.; Dittert, L.W.; Griffen, W.O., Jr.; Doluisio, J.T.: Pharmacokinetics of pentobarbital after intravenous and oral administration. J. Pharmacokinet. Biopharm. *1:* 5–15 (1973).

40 Walle, T.; Fagan, T.; Walle, K.U.; Oexmann, M.-J.; Conradi, E.C.; Gaffney, T.E.: Food-induced increase in propranolol bioavailability – relationship to protein and effects on metabolites. Clin. Pharmacol. Ther. *30:* 790–795 (1981).

41 Welling, P.G.: How food and fluid affect drug absorption. Postgrad. Med. *62:* 73–82 (1977).

42 Wåhlin-Boll, E.; Melander, A.; Sartor, G.; Scherstén, B.: Influence of food intake on the absorption and effect of glipizide in diabetics and in healthy subjects. Eur. J. clin. Pharmacol. *18:* 279–283 (1980).

A. Melander, MD, Division of Clinical Pharmacology, Lund University Health Sciences Center, S–240 10 Dalby (Sweden)

Wld Rev. Nutr. Diet., vol. 43, pp. 45–59 (Karger, Basel 1984)

Environmental Influences on Drug Biotransformations in Humans

Alvito P. Alvares[1]

Department of Pharmacology, Uniformed Services University, Bethesda, Md., USA

A major problem for both pharmacologists and physicians concerns the large degree of interindividual variation in rates of drug disposition that occur among normal subjects, as well as patients, in response to a particular drug. Such interindividual variations have been demonstrated for many drugs. The magnitude of interindividual variations in rate of elimination of a drug, in a group of subjects administered the same dosage, can range from 4-fold to 40-fold. Such interindividual variations in drug disposition may determine why a drug may cause a pronounced pharmacological response or even a toxic response in one individual and little or no therapeutic response in another patient. In recent years, numerous drugs with low therapeutic indices have been introduced, thereby increasing the risk of toxicity when these drugs are administered to slow or fast metabolizers. Epidemiological studies have shown diversities in the incidence of neoplasms between various populations. The differences that are found may be partly due to changes in environmental factors which protect the host against the effect of a particular chemical carcinogen. Many chemical carcinogens are metabolized to their active metabolites by enzymes localized in the endoplasmic reticulum, which also metabolize or biotransform drugs and other foreign chemicals.

In addition to disease states, variability in rates of drug metabolism in man is caused by genetic as well as by environmental factors. Despite

[1] I thank *Jean Bartlett* for her secretarial help in the preparation of this manuscript.

numerous studies, the relative role of genetics and the environment in regulating human drug metabolism is not known for certain. Studies by *Vesell and Page* [1, 2] and by *Alexanderson* et al. [3] have demonstrated that genetic factors play an important role in controlling the rate of human drug metabolism. An approach for assessing the role of the environment in regulating the metabolism of a drug is to study the metabolism of the drug in the same subject on several occasions. Any change in the rate of drug metabolism that occurs in an individual when the drug is administered on different occasions may be attributed to changes in the subject's external environment and/or physiological factors (internal environment). In a recent study, we studied the effect of the environment in controlling human drug metabolism by administering phenylbutazone, antipyrine or phenacetin to 7 normal subjects (non-smokers who were not ingesting any drugs or other known enzyme inducers or inhibitors) on five occasions at 6-week intervals [4]. In these subjects no attempt was made to control the life-styles or diets of the subjects during the course of the study. Moderate variability occurred in the metabolism of phenylbutazone, a drug which has a long plasma elimination rate. Intraindividual differences in the plasma half-lives of antipyrine were greater than for phenylbutazone. When the analgesic, phenacetin, was administered to the same subjects on five occasions, intraindividual differences in the plasma half-lives of phenacetin were more marked than for antipyrine or phenylbutazone. The plasma half-life of phenacetin varied from a 30% range in subject A to 100% in subjects B and D (fig. 1). The mean change in the plasma half-life of phenacetin from the lowest to the highest value in each individual was 63% for the 7 subjects studied (fig. 1). The smallest area under the phenacetin plasma concentration-time curve (0→7 h) was 19 $\mu g \cdot min \cdot ml^{-1}$ (subject B) and the largest was 1,110 $\mu g \cdot min \cdot ml^{-1}$ (subject D). These and other studies with theophylline [5] indicate that unidentified environmental factors play an important role in regulating human drug metabolism.

In recent years man has been exposed to increasingly large amounts of environmental chemicals and many of these substances stimulate or inhibit drug disposition. Examples of stimulators of drug metabolism in animals include halogenated hydrocarbon pesticides, polycyclic aromatic hydrocarbons, herbicides, occupational exposure to chemicals, food additives, tobacco smoke, and normal constituents of food. Environmental chemicals which inhibit drug metabolism include organophosphorous insecticides, certain heavy metals, carbon monoxide and aliphatic chlorinated compounds.

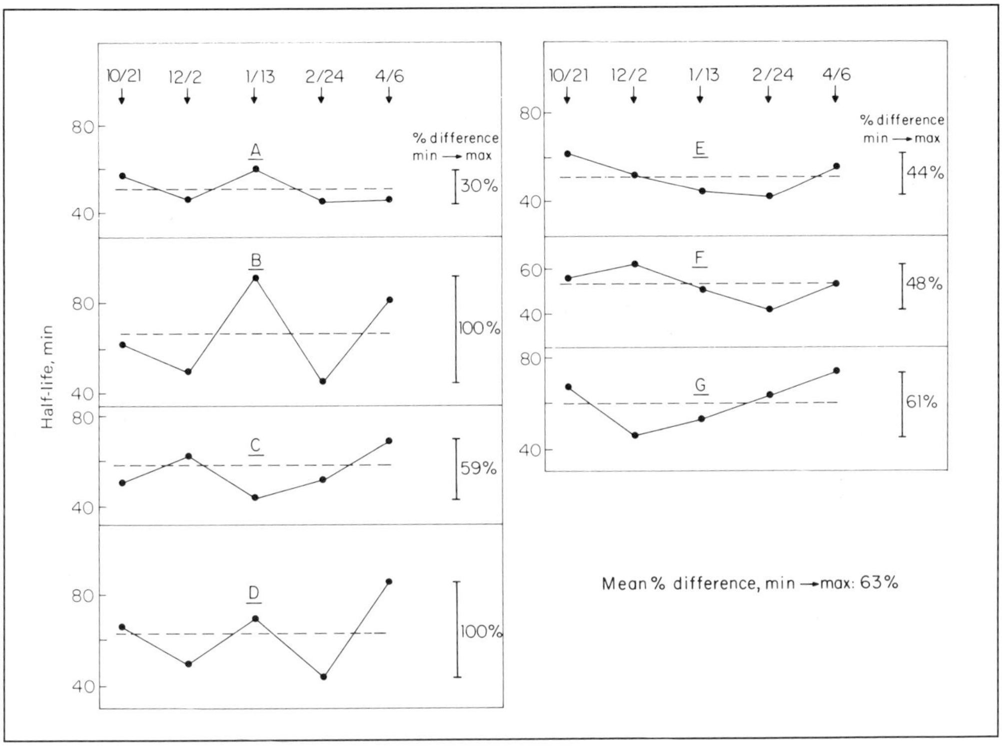

Fig. 1. Intraindividual variations in plasma half-lives of phenacetin in normal subjects. Phenacetin, 900 mg was administered orally to 7 subjects at 6-week intervals on the dates indicated at the top of the figure. The dashed line represents the mean of five half-life values determined for each individual. The percent difference between the maximum and minimum half-life of each subjects was calculated as follows: $\left(\frac{\text{max}}{\text{min}} - 1\right) \times 100$ [from ref. 4].

Alterations in Drug Metabolism Induced by Cigarette Smoke

The interactions of cigarette smoking and drug disposition is of great social and medical importance, and smoking thus offers the potential for causing a high incidence of altered drug metabolism. The most common effect of smoking on drug disposition in man is an increase in biotransformation rates, consistent with induction of drug-metabolizing enzymes. Among those drugs for which dispositional characteristics are altered are phenacetin, imipramine, theophylline, and antipyrine. Hepatic oxidative metabolism of each is apparently enhanced presumably due to polycyclic aromatic hydrocarbons, such as benzo(a)pyrene, present in cigarette smoke. These hydrocarbons are well-known inducers of hepatic microsomal monooxygenases in rodents as well as man.

The interaction of theophylline and tobacco smoke is one of the most chemically significant effects of smoking because of the low therapeutic index of this drug and the great variability in disposition rates among patients. *Jenne* et al. [6] found theophylline half-lives of about 4 h in young smokers and about 7 h in non-smokers. *Hunt* et al. [7] showed that smokers showed about twice the metabolic clearance rates for theophylline compared to non-smokers. A marked increase in clearance of caffeine by smokers, when compared to non-smokers, has been observed by *Parsons and Neims* [8]. This increased clearance may contribute to the higher consumption of coffee reported to occur among cigarette smokers. The inductive effects of cigarette smoking on the biotransformation of a widely used drug in man was first studied extensively by *Pantuck* et al. [9]. Following the administration of a single oral dose of phenacetin to smokers and non-smokers, it was found that the plasma levels of phenacetin were considerably lower in cigarette smokers than in non-smokers (table I). Interestingly, the plasma concentrations of N-acetyl-*p*-aminophenol, its major metabolite, and the plasma half-life of phenacetin were similar in smokers and in non-smokers. The authors concluded that cigarette smoking markedly decreases the bioavailability of phenacetin and suggested that this decrease was due to the enhancement of phenacetin metabolism during its first pass through the liver and/or increased metabolism of the analgesic in the intestine of the smokers.

With large segments of the population engaged in smoking tobacco, there is a potential for a high incidence of altered drug disposition and

Table I. Plasma levels of phenacetin in cigarette smokers and non-smokers

Subjects	Phenacetin in plasma (μg/ml) at intervals after administration (h)			
	1 h	2 h	3.5 h	5 h
Non-smokers	0.81 ± 0.20	2.24 ± 0.73	0.39 ± 0.13	0.12 ± 0.04
Smokers	0.33 ± 0.23	0.48 ± 0.28	0.09 ± 0.04	0.02 ± 0.01

9 cigarette smokers and 9 non-smokers were administered a single dose of 900 mg of phenacetin orally. Each value represents the mean ± SE for 9 subjects [from ref. 9].

therapeutic response. The extent of tobacco usage and its effect on disposition of certain drugs requires that smoking status may be an important determinant in drug action and interaction.

Alterations in Drug Metabolism Induced by Ethanol

Ethyl alcohol, one of the more widespread environmental chemicals of human intake, is the only one regularly consumed in multigram quantities. Ethanol directly interferes with the pharmacological action of many drugs, particularly neuropharmacologically active drugs. However, there is also an indirect interaction relating to the effects of ethanol ingestion on the metabolism of the drugs. In the latter respect, acute and chronic effects of ethanol are usually opposite. Although there are some exceptions, generally, an acute dose of ethanol inhibits the biotransformation of drugs metabolized by the liver monooxygenase system, whereas chronic consumption enhances drug metabolism, often because of the induction of liver microsomal enzymes.

The presence of ethanol modifies the response to drugs. The acute oral administration of ethanol results in a prolongation of the half-life of pentobarbital and meprobamate from the blood in humans (table II). The inter-

Table II. Effect of acute ethanol administration on plasma elimination rates of pentobarbital and meprobamate

Subject	Pentobarbital $t_{1/2}$, h		Meprobamate $t_{1/2}$, h	
	control	after ethanol	control	after ethanol
1	39	76	8.9	43.0
2	28	56	8.6	29.5
3	21	50	8.7	28.7
4	31	53	7.4	13.7
$\bar{x}$	30	59	8.4	28.7

4 volunteer subjects were given 6 mg/kg pentoarbital or 12–15 mg/kg meprobamate. Ethanol was administered orally at an initial dosage of 1 g/kg, followed by 24 g every 2 h [from ref. 10].

action of ethanol with barbiturates represents a particular danger. The lethal dose for barbiturates is nearly 50% lower in the presence of alcohol than it is when the drug is used alone [11]. It has indeed been found that ethanol inhibits the metabolism of a variety of drugs in vitro. These in vitro effects may explain the observation that in vivo, simultaneous administration of ethanol and drugs slows the rate of drug metabolism.

Apparent increases in the metabolism and clearance of some drugs have been noted following chronic ethanol ingestion. In animals, chronic administration of ethanol causes proliferation of hepatic smooth endoplasmic reticulum, and increases in the cytochrome P-450 system which is involved in the oxidative metabolism of drugs [review in ref. 12]. The effects of chronic ethanol administration to man on the plasma elimination rate of antipyrine in 6 normal subjects are shown in table III. Although the mean half-life of antipyrine decreased by about 25%, it is of interest to note the interindividual variation in the inducibility of the test drug. Subject 5 did not show any change in plasma half-life of antipyrine. Such interindividual variations have also been observed by other investigators, using such classical enzyme inducers as phenobarbital. Other studies have shown that chronic administration of ethanol to rats or man results in an increase in the rate of metabolism of pentobarbital, meprobamate, aminopyrine, tolbutamide, warfarin, and theophylline. Although ethanol may interact with the

Table III. Effect of chronic ethanol administration on antipyrine metabolism

Subject	Antipyrine $t_{1/2}$		Reduction in $t_{1/2}$, %
	before ethanol	after ethanol	
1	11.0	8.0	27.3
2	16.5	10.5	36.4
3	30.0	19.0	36.7
4	10.5	9.0	14.3
5	12.0	11.5	4.2
6	14.0	12.0	14.3
$\bar{x}$	15.7	11.7	25.5

6 healthy subjects received 95% ethanol, 1 ml/kg/day for 21 days. On days 1 and 21, antipyrine, 18 mg/kg, was administered and plasma half-life of the drug was determined [from ref. 13].

microsomal enzyme systems which oxidize drugs and may be partially metabolized by this enzyme system, it should be noted that ethanol is metabolized primarily by the cytosolic enzyme alcohol dehydrogenase, and to a lesser extent by catalase in peroxisomes.

Effect of Non-Nutrient Dietary Contaminants on Drug Metabolism

Substances present in food that may influence the metabolism of drugs include macronutrients (carbohydrate, protein, fat), trace substances important to human health (vitamins, trace metals, etc.) and numerous non-nutrient, lipid-soluble foreign chemicals. Although the latter very diverse group of substances has not been well characterized, its presence in foods is receiving increasingly more attention. Since humans receive most of their exposure to exogenous chemicals through diet, it is important to determine the effects of these non-nutrients on the metabolism of drugs, and other environmental pollutants.

Safrole (4-allyl-1,2-methylenedioxybenzene) is a natural plant constituent, found in oil of sassafras and certain other essential oils. It is a member of the methylenedioxybenzene group of compounds, many of which (e.g. piperonyl butoxide) are extensively used as insecticide synergists. A major source of human exposure to safrole is through the consumption of spices, such as nutmeg, cinnamon and black pepper, in which it is a constituent. Safrole is also present in root beer, and has been used as an additive in chewing gum, toothpaste, and soaps. Safrole has also been found to be a weak hepatocarcinogen. Its metabolism gives rise to intermediates capable of covalent binding with DNA and protein. The parent compound and its metabolites have been found to be mutagenic [review in ref. 14].

In hepatic as well as non-hepatic tissues, the terminal oxidase which oxidatively metabolizes drugs and other foreign chemicals is a family of hemoproteins collectively known as cytochrome P-450. Safrole, as a substrate for the hepatic monooxygenases, binds to cytochrome P-450, and in the presence of NADPH and oxygen, is transformed to reactive intermediates. Its binding properties with cytochrome P-450 cause a decrease in the concentration of free cytochrome P-450 and a concomitant loss of mixed function oxidase activity [15]. However, like many inhibitors, safrole and isosafrole on chronic administration induce microsomal cytochrome P-450. Recent studies have led to the isolation and purification from isosafrole-pretreated rats of a unique form of hepatic cytochrome P-450 [16].

The biological and clinical significance of this new hemeprotein induced by this non-nutrient remains to be determined.

Polycyclic aromatic hydrocarbons are experimentally well established carcinogens. Man may be exposed to these carcinogens through smoking, coal-tar dermatologic preparations, as products of incomplete combustion, and through smoked and charcoal-broiled foods. It has recently been reported that pyrolysis products of proteins and amino acids are highly mutagenic [17]. Although pyrolysates of tryptophan, glutamic acid, lysine, ornithine, and serine all show very high mutagenic activity with *Salmonella typhimurium,* they are not effective as inducers of carcinogen-metabolizing species of cytochrome P-450. One group of food additives, namely phenolic antioxidants, alters microsomal monooxygenases. The antioxidant butylated hydroxyanisole (BHA) has been found to exert a protective effect against chemical carcinogens [18].

Since the polycyclic aromatic hydrocarbon benzo(a)pyrene is a constituent of charcoal-broiled beef [19] and since charcoal-broiled beef is eaten by large numbers of people, it was of interest to determine if meat cooked in this manner would affect drug metabolism in man. The following summarizes our studies on the effect of charcoal broiling of meat on the metabolic disposition of phenacetin, antipyrine, and theophylline in man [20–22]. In these studies 900 mg of phenacetin was administered to healthy subjects after they had been fed (1) a control diet for several days, (2) a charcoal-broiled beef diet for 4 days, and (3) a control diet for an additional 7 days. During the control diet periods, the meat was cooked over burning charcoal with aluminum foil placed between the meat and the burning charcoal. During the second experimental period, the meat was cooked directly over the burning charcoal. Details of this study are given elsewhere [21, 22]. Feeding the charcoal-broiled beef diet for 4 days markedly lowered the plasma concentrations of phenacetin (table IV). In data not shown, the charcoal-broiled beef diet did not change the plasma half-life of phenacetin, nor did it have a significant effect on the plasma concentrations of its major metabolite, N-acetyl-*p*-aminophenol. Thus, the ratios of metabolite/parent compound levels were markedly elevated when subjects were fed the charcoal-broiled diet. These results strongly suggest that a charcoal-broiled beef diet greatly increases the metabolism of phenacetin during its first pass through the liver and/or in the gastrointestinal tract.

Similar protocols were used to determine whether eating a charcoal-broiled beef diet would influence the metabolism of antipyrine, or the bronchodilator theophylline. As shown in table V, feeding the charcoal-broiled

Table IV. Effect of a diet containing charcoal-broiled beef on the plasma concentration of phenacetin in man

Diet	Plasma concentration of phenacetin (ng/ml) at intervals (h) after its administration					
	1 h	2 h	3 h	4 h	5 h	7 h
Control (1st time)	1,328 ± 481	925 ± 166	313 ± 60	149 ± 27	66 ± 14	17 ± 4
Charcoal-broiled beef	319 ± 90	163 ± 32	74 ± 17	34 ± 9	15 ± 4	7 ± 2
Control (2nd time)	1,827 ± 661	623 ± 128	271 ± 76	99 ± 24	40 ± 11	14 ± 4

900 mg of phenacetin was administered orally after each dietary regimen, and plasma was analyzed for phenacetin at various intervals after the dose. Each value represents the mean ± SE for 9 subjects [from ref. 20, 21].

Table V. Effect of a diet containing charcoal-broiled beef on antipyrine and theophylline metabolism in man

Diet	Antipyrine		Theophylline	
	half-life h	metabolic clearance rate ml/min	half-life h	metabolic clearance rate ml/min
Control (1st time)	13.7 ± 1.3	45.8 ± 4.2	6.0 ± 0.5	69.8 ± 6.3
Charcoal-broiled beef	10.7 ± 1.2	63.2 ± 6.4	4.7 ± 0.4	90.9 ± 9.3
Control (2nd time)	13.3 ± 1.1	47.5 ± 4.5	6.4 ± 0.7	69.1 ± 1.1

Antipyrine (1.8 mg/kg) or theophylline (5 mg/kg) was administered orally after 3–4 days on control diet, 3–4 days on charcoal-broiled beef diet, and again at 5–6 days on the control diet. Each value represents the mean ± SE for 8 subjects [from ref. 22].

beef diet to normal subjects decreased the plasma half-life of antipyrine by 22% and increased its apparent metabolic clearance rate by 38%. Feeding this diet decreased the theophylline half-life by 22% and increased its apparent metabolic clearance rate by 30% (table V). With both test drugs, there was no significant effect on the apparent volume of distribution. These data demonstrate that a short period of human ingestion of only moderate amounts of charcoal-broiled beef significantly enhances the hepatic oxidations of the above test drugs. It would be of interest to determine if these observations extend to other foods which may contain polycyclic aromatic hydrocarbons such as smoked foods, or to psoriatic patients being treated with coal-tar-containing ointments. The effects of charcoal-broiled meat on phenacetin metabolism are similar to those reported (table I) for cigarette smokers.

Effects of Dietary Protein and Carbohydrate on Drug Metabolism

Of all the dietary manipulations, the extreme form, that of starvation, would be expected to produce the most marked pharmacokinetic alteration. Studies by *Reidenberg* [23] and *Reidenberg and Vesell* [24] have shown that fasting produces no major changes in rates of metabolism of sulfisoxazole, isoniazid, procaine, antipyrine, and tolbutamide. These conclusions were further substantiated by a study of female patients with confirmed, classical anorexia nervosa. These latter patients had normal antipyrine pharmacokinetics [25] when these values were corrected for body weight.

The most dramatic changes in drug metabolism in humans occur when macronutrient composition of the diet is altered. The effects of isocaloric substitution of carbohydrate for protein was studied over a time period of controlled dietary intake totalling 4 weeks [26, 27]. 6 normal subjects were placed first on a high protein-low carbohydrate diet for 2 weeks followed by a high carbohydrate-low protein diet for 2 weeks. During this 4-week experimental period, the amount of protein was decreased from 44% in the high protein diet to 10% in the low protein diet. Concomitantly, the amount of total calories represented by carbohydrates doubled from 35 to 70%. The amount of total calories represented by fat remained constant in the two diets at approximately 20%. For each subject, antipyrine and theophylline plasma half-lives were determined on days 10 and 14, respectively, of each 2-week experimental period. Details of the experimental protocol have been previously described [27]. As shown in figure 2, in all 6 subjects studied the theophylline half-life was greater when the subjects were on a high carbohydrate-low protein diet, than when the same subjects were placed on the high protein-low carbohydrate diet. The mean theophylline half-life of 5.23 h on the high protein diet was significantly different from the mean half-life of 7.62 h on the low protein diet. Similar results were obtained when antipyrine was used as the test drug. These data demonstrate that a change in macronutrient composition of carbohydrate and protein can cause significant changes in the plasma elimination rates of antipyrine and theophylline.

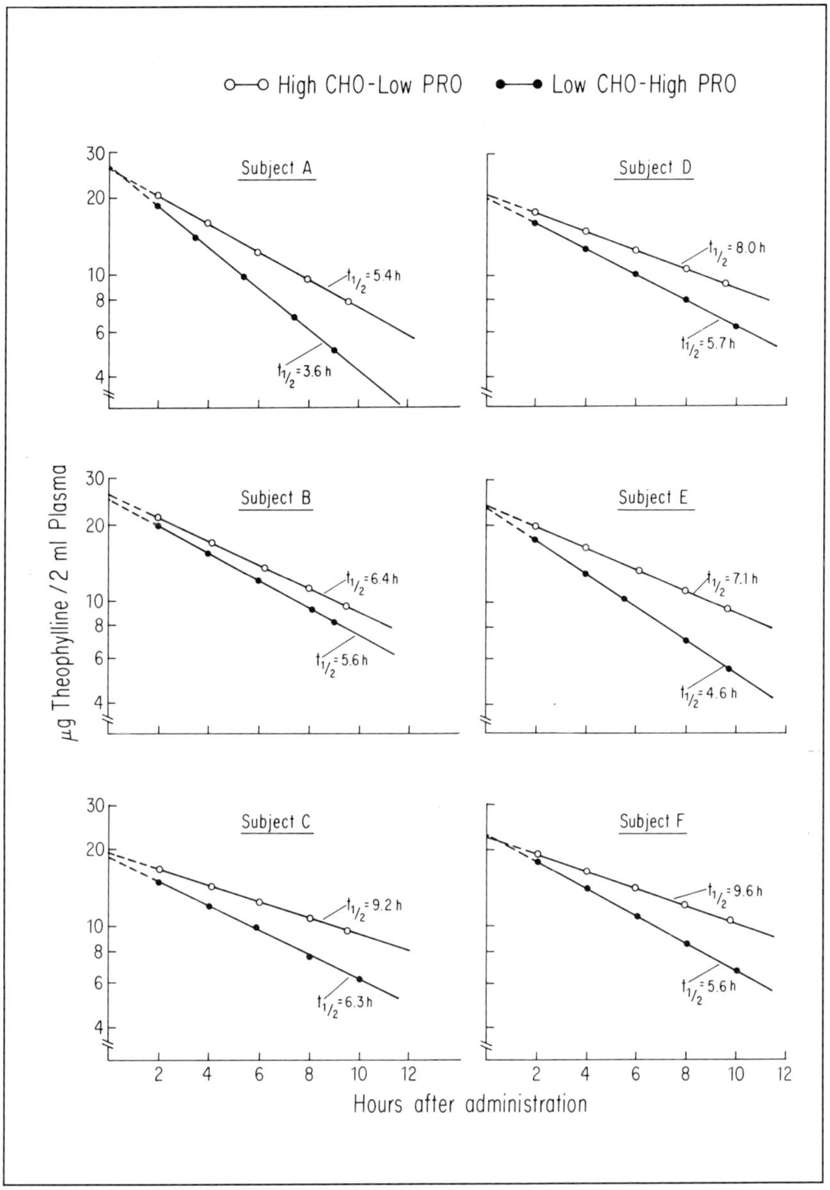

Fig. 2. Decline of theophylline in the plasma of 6 normal subjects fed low carbohydrate-high protein tests diets followed by high carbohydrate-low protein test diets. The subjects were maintained on each test diet for 14 days, and theophylline, 5 mg/kg, was administered orally as a single dose on day 14 of each test diet period [from ref. 27].

The nutritional-pharmacological interactions may have considerable importance in vast segments of the population who undertake weight-reducing regimens; in large numbers of postoperative patients who receive glucose intravenously as a sole form of nourishment, and in large numbers of patients whose disease processes (i.e. diabetes, atherosclerosis, etc.) require significant nutritional restrictions. In those subjects, who change their dietary patterns in ways similar to those described above, drug dosage may also have to be changed to prevent toxic or non-therapeutic blood levels of the drug.

Effects of Vegetables on Drug Metabolism

Cruciferous vegetables including Brussels sprouts, cabbage, and cauliflower are inducers of hepatic monooxygenases in rodents [28, 29]. From these vegetables three indoles with inducing activity have been identified. These are indole-3-acetonitrile, indole-3-carbinol, and 3,3′-diindolylmethane [30]. Other compounds found in plants also have inducing activity. A few flavones, such as 5,6,7,8,4′-pentamethoxyflavone (tangeretin) and 4,5,7,8,3,4′-hexamethoxyflavone (nobiletin) present in citrus fruits induce aryl hydrocarbon hydroxylase in rats [31].

Studies in normal subjects fed test diets containing Brussels sprouts and cabbage showed a small but statistically significant decrease in mean antipyrine plasma half-life and an increase in the mean metabolic clearance rate. When phenacetin was used as the test drug in the same subjects, the average plasma concentration of phenacetin was decreased by 34–67% when measured repeatedly during the period 0.5–7 h after the administration of the drug [32]. Although these studies indicate that certain vegetables may enhance the metabolism of test drugs, recent studies [33] on Indo-Pakistani immigrants in England have shown that the metabolic clearance rate of antipyrine among lactovegetarians was significantly slower than in the subjects who ate meat regularly. The apparent effect of meat in this study could relate to the observed difference in protein intake, fat intake or both. Daily protein intake was significantly lower amongst vegetarians, and this could account for the differences in rates of metabolism of the test drug. These data have particular significance, since large segments of the population in certain Third World countries, and smaller segments in the Western countries are vegetarians. In these individuals, it is likely that lower average daily doses of drugs metabolized by hepatic oxidation would be required.

Activation of Monooxygenases by Food Contaminants

Treatment of animals or exposure of humans to certain drugs and other foreign chemicals induces the synthesis of hepatic monooxygenases. At least several hours is required for the induction of measurable increases in monooxygenase activity, and these inductive properties can be inhibited in vivo by inhibitors of protein synthesis. More recently, it has been found that the oxidation of various drugs and chemical carcinogens by hepatic cytochrome P-450-dependent monooxygenases can be stimulated in vitro by the addition of certain foreign chemicals to the incubation medium. This activation process, in contrast to enzyme induction, does not depend on the synthesis of new enzyme protein. *Kapitulnik* et al. [34] and *Buening* et al. [35] have shown that certain flavones, naturally occurring compounds found in several plant species, stimulated the hydroxylation of benzo(a)pyrene, zoxazolamine and antipyrine and the metabolism of aflatoxin B_1 and benzo(a)pyrene 7,8-dihydrodiol to mutagens by human liver. More recently, *Lasker* et al. [36] demonstrated severalfold stimulation of zoxazolamine metabolism in vivo following the injection of neonatal rats with flavone. These data are highly significant since human ingestion of such metabolic activators present in the diet or in the environment could cause immediate increases in the rates of metabolism of drugs, carcinogens and other lipid-soluble chemicals. However, it is yet to be determined if humans would normally ingest enough of the activators to cause stimulation of drug or carcinogen metabolism.

In summary, marked variations in responsiveness to drugs occur in man. Such interindividual variations can be partly attributed to genetic factors. However, man is exposed to a variety of chemicals in his environment, and some of these have been shown to alter drug biotransformations as well. Besides the inadvertent exposure to environmental chemicals, diet is a major point of direct contact between man and his external environment. Studies described above show that macronutrients, micronutrients and non-nutrients in the diet can influence drug disposition. The ingestion of alcohol can also alter rates of drug metabolism. Another common social habit, namely cigarette smoking, has been shown to enhance the in vivo metabolism of drugs. It should also be noted that occupational exposure to enzyme inducers or inhibitors may be another environmental factor that may alter the pharmacologic action of drugs and other foreign chemicals. Thus, either alone or operating in concert with still other factors, dietary alterations could appreciably change the metabolic clearance of drugs.

References

1 Vesell, E.S.; Page, J.G.: Genetic control of drug levels in man: Antipyrine. Science *161:* 72–73 (1968).

2 Vesell, E.S.; Page, J.G.: Genetic control of the phenobarbitol-induced shortening of plasma antipyrine half-lives in man. J. clin. Invest. *48:* 2202–2209 (1969).

3 Alexanderson, B.; Evans, A.P.; Sjöqvist, F.: Steady-state plasma levels of nortriptyline in twins: influence of genetic factors and drug therapy. Br. med. J. *74:* 764–768 (1969).

4 Alvares, A.P.; Kappas, A.; Eiseman, J.L.; Anderson, K.E.; Pantuck, C.B.; Pantuck, E.J.; Hsiao, K.-C.; Garland, W.A.; Conney, A.H.: Intraindividual variation in drug disposition. Clin. Pharmacol. Ther. *26:* 407–419 (1979).

5 Walson, P.D.; Strunk, R.C.; Taussig, L.M.: Intrapatient variability in theophylline kinetics. J. Pediat. *91:* 321–324 (1977).

6 Jenne, J.; Nagasawa, H.; McHugh, R.M.; Macdonald, F.; Wyse, E.: Decreased theophylline half-life in cigarette smokers. Life Sci. *17:* 195–198 (1975).

7 Hunt, S.N.; Jusko, W.J.; Yurchak, A.M.: Effect of cigarette smoking on theophylline disposition. Clin. Pharmacol. Ther. *19:* 546–551 (1976).

8 Parsons, W.D.; Neims, A.H.: Effect of smoking on caffeine clearance. Clin. Pharmacol. Ther. *24:* 40–45 (1978).

9 Pantuck, E.J.; Hsiao, K.-C.; Maggio, A.; Nakamura, A.; Kuntzman, R.; Conney, A.H.: Effect of cigarette smoking on phenacetin metabolism. Clin. Pharmacol. Ther. *15:* 9–17 (1974).

10 Rubin, E.; Gang, H.; Misra, P.S.; Lieber, C.S.: Inhibition of drug metabolism by acute ethanol intoxication: a hepatic microsomal inhibition. Am. J. Med. *49:* 801–806 (1970).

11 Bogan, J.; Smith, M.: Analytical investigation of barbiturate poisoning: description, methods and a survey of results. J. forens. Sci. *7:* 37–45 (1967).

12 Lieber, C.S.: Interaction of ethanol with drug toxicity. Am. J. Gastroent. *74:* 313–320 (1980).

13 Vesell, E.S.; Page, J.G.; Passananti, G.T.: Genetic and environmental factors affecting ethanol metabolism in man. Clin. Pharmacol. Ther. *12:* 192–201 (1971).

14 Ioannides, C.; Delaforge, M.; Parke, D.V.: Safrole: its metabolism, carcinogenicity and interactions with cytochrome P-450. Fd. Cosmet. Toxicol. *19:* 657–666 (1981).

15 Anders, M.W.: Inhibition of microsomal drug metabolism by methylenedioxybenzenes. Biochem. Pharmacol. *17:* 2367–2370 (1968).

16 Ryan, D.E.; Thomas, P.E.; Levin, W.: Hepatic microsomal cytochrome P-450 from rats treated with isosafrole. J. biol. Chem. *255:* 7941–7955 (1980).

17 Nebert, D.W.; Bigelow, S.W.; Okey, A.B.; Yahagi, T.; Mori, Y.; Nagao, M.; Sugimura, T.: Pyrolysis products from amino acids and proteins: highest mutagenicity requires cytochrome P_1-450. Proc. natn. Acad. Sci. USA *76:* 5929–5933 (1979).

18 Wattenberg, L.W.: Effects of dietary constituents on the metabolism of chemical carcinogens. Cancer Res. *35:* 3326–3331 (1975).

19 Lijinsky, W.; Shubik, P.: Benzo(a)pyrene and other polynuclear hydrocarbons in charcoal-broiled meat. Science *145:* 53–55 (1964).

20 Pantuck, E.J.; Hsiao, K.-C.; Conney, A.H.; Garland, W.; Kappas, A.; Anderson, K.; Alvares, A.P.: Effect of charcoal-broiled beef on phenacetin metabolism in man. Science *194:* 1055–1057 (1976).

21 Conney, A.H.; Pantuck, E.J.; Hsiao, K.-C.; Garland, W.A.; Anderson, K.E.; Alvares, A.P.; Kappas, A.: Enhanced phenacetin metabolism in human subjects fed charcoal-broiled beef. Clin. Pharmacol. Ther. *20:* 633–642 (1976).
22 Kappas, A.; Alvares, A.P.; Anderson, K.E.; Pantuck, E.J.; Pantuck, C.B.; Chang, R.; Conney, A.H.: Effect of charcoal-broiled beef on antipyrine and theophylline metabolism. Clin. Pharmacol. Ther. *23:* 445–450 (1978).
23 Reidenberg, M.M.: Obesity and fasting-effects on drug metabolism and drug action in man. Clin. Pharmacol. Ther. *22:* 729–734 (1977).
24 Reidenberg, M.M.; Vesell, E.S.: Unaltered metabolism of antipyrine and tolbutamide in fasting man. Clin. Pharmacol. Ther. *17:* 650–656 (1975).
25 Bakke, O.M.; Aanderud, S.; Syversen, G.; Bassoe, H.H.; Myking, O.: Antipyrine metabolism in anorexia nervosa. Br. J. clin. Pharmacol. *5:* 341–343 (1978).
26 Alvares, A.P.; Anderson, K.E.; Conney, A.H.; Kappas, A.: Interactions between nutritional factors and drug biotransformations in man. Proc. natn. Acad. Sci. USA *73:* 2501–2504 (1976).
27 Kappas, A.; Anderson, K.E.; Conney, A.H.; Alvares, A.P.: Influence of dietary protein and carbohydrate on antipyrine and theophylline metabolism in man. Clin. Pharmacol. Ther. *20:* 643–653 (1976).
28 Wattenberg, L.W.: Studies of polycyclic hydrocarbon hydroxylases of the intestine possibly related to cancer. Effect of diet on benzpyrene hydroxylase activity. Cancer *28:* 99–102 (1971).
29 Pantuck, E.J.; Hsiao, K.-C.; Loub, W.D.; Wattenberg, L.W.; Kuntzman, R.; Conney, A.H.: Stimulatory effect of vegetables on intestinal drug metabolism in the rat. J. Pharmac. exp. Ther. *198:* 278–283 (1976).
30 Loub, W.D.; Wattenberg, L.W.; Davis, D.W.: Aryl hydrocarbon hydroxylase induction in rat tissues by naturally occurring indoles of cruciferous plants. J. natn. Cancer Inst. *54:* 985–988 (1975).
31 Wattenberg, L.W.; Page, M.A.; Leong, J.L.: Induction of increased benzpyrene hydroxylase activity by flavones and related compounds. Cancer Res. *28:* 934–937 (1968).
32 Pantuck, E.J.; Pantuck, C.B.; Garland, W.A.; Min, B.H.; Wattenberg, L.W.; Anderson, K.E.; Kappas, A.; Conney, A.H.: Stimulatory effects of Brussels sprouts and cabbage on human drug metabolism. Clin. Pharmacol. Ther. *25:* 88–95 (1979).
33 Mucklow, J.C.; Caraher, M.T.; Henderson, D.B.; Chapman, P.H.; Roberts, D.F.; Rawlins, M.D.: The relationship between individual dietary constituents and antipyrine metabolism in Indo-Pakistani immigrants to Britain. Br. J. clin. Pharmacol. *13:* 481–486 (1982).
34 Kapitulnik, J.; Poppers, P.J.; Buening, M.K.; Fortner, J.G.; Conney, A.H.: Activation of monooxygenases in human liver by 7,8-benzoflavone. Clin. Pharmacol. Ther. *22:* 475–484 (1977).
35 Buening, M.K.; Chang, R.L.; Huang, M.-T.; Fortner, J.G.; Wood, A.W.; Conney, A.H.: Activation and inhibition of benzo(a)pyrene and aflatoxin B_1 metabolism in human liver microsomes by naturally occurring flavonoids. Cancer Res. *41:* 67–72 (1981).
36 Lasker, J.M.; Huang, M.-T.; Conney, A.H.: In vivo activation of zoxazolamine metabolism by flavone. Science *216:* 1419–1421 (1982).

A.P. Alvares, PhD, Department of Pharmacology,
Uniformed Services University, Bethesda, MD 20814 (USA)

Wld Rev. Nutr. Diet., vol. 43, pp. 60–79 (Karger, Basel 1984)

Maternal Drug Use: Evaluation of Risks to Breast-Fed Infants

A. Kirksey, S.M. Groziak

Department of Food and Nutrition, Purdue University, West Lafayette, Ind., USA

The recent dramatic increase in developed countries in breast-feeding for extended periods of time coupled with the current widespread use of medications leads to some concern about the well-being of breast-fed infants. Almost all drugs pass into human milk and consideration of their benefits to the mother must be carefully weighed against their risks to the infant. The potential harm of a particular drug to the breast-fed infant is related both to the complex mechanism of milk synthesis and secretion and to the mode of passage of the drug from plasma into milk.

Mammary Cell and Milk Synthesis

Mammary cells are desmosomally connected, uninuclear, and change from cuboidal shape prior to prolactin stimulation to cylindrical just prior to milk secretion (fig. 1). The vascular system surrounding the cells is extensive with a thin band of connective tissue, the alveolar basal lamina, separating the capillaries and cells [1]. Cells progressively extend towards the lumen as synthesized substances (fat, protein and lactose) accumulate and rise toward the apical membrane. In the process of milk synthesis several opportunities exist for drugs to be excreted into milk and to be bound to milk constituents. Casein, lactalbumin and lactoglobulin are synthesized on rough endoplasmic reticulum and then are transported to the Golgi apparatus where they condense into granules which may be released into the cytoplasm and migrate to the apical membrane for merocrine secretion. More commonly, Golgi vesicles migrate to the apex of the cell to release their contents into the lumen [2]. This is reverse pinocytosis or apocrine secre-

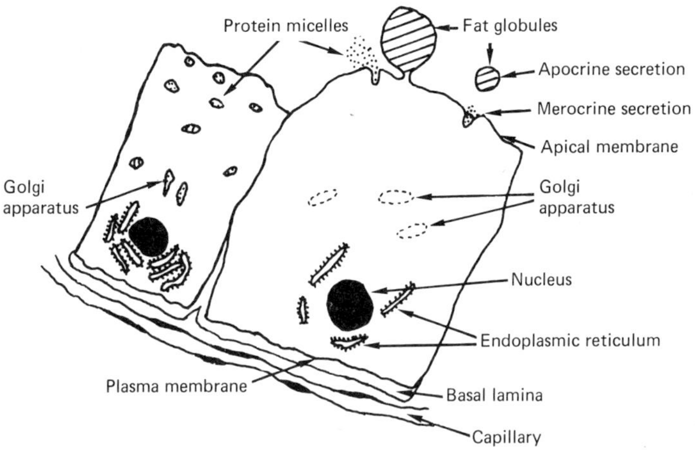

Fig. 1. Schematic drawing of mammary glandular cells in secreting phase.

tion whereby the apical part of the glandular cell is released along with the secreted protein. Drugs may be excreted into milk by binding to these proteins. Following fat synthesis, lipids coalesce and acquire a lipoprotein coating as they migrate toward the apical membrane for apocrine secretion [3]. Drugs may bind to the lipoprotein coating or be trapped in the fat globule during its formation. Synthesis of lactose, which is catalyzed by α-lactalbumin within the Golgi apparatus, leads to osmotic swelling followed by its release via both apocrine and merocrine processes.

Milk Secretion and Composition

The major stimulus for milk production and secretion is prolactin. The release of this hormone is highest under the stimulus of sucking and, therefore, most milk is synthesized either during or shortly after the nursing period. Hence drugs excreted into milk should reflect simultaneous plasma levels [3]. Human milk output ranges from an average of 600–1,000 ml/day and can be controlled by the mother since it is proportional to the nursing time allowed. However, little control can be exercised over the changes in milk composition which occur diurnally and with the progression of lactation. Each major phase of lactation (colostrum, transitional and mature milk) represents differences in fat content and pH [4]. Colostrum has a high specific gravity (SG) and pH but low fat content compared to mature milk [1]. Fat content shows diurnal fluctuation, is highest in the early morning, and increases from fore to hind milk at each feeding. Milk composition, pH and SG influence the extent to which a drug passes from plasma into milk.

Mode of Passage of Drugs into Milk

Drugs filter into milk across a series of structural barriers: capillary wall, interstitial fluid and mammary cell basal lamina and plasma membrane [5] (fig. 1). Only non-protein bound pharmacons cross the capillary wall and this is by endothelial pores via diffusion, filtration or reverse pinocytosis. The speed of transport depends upon molecular weight, pK_a, solubility, and polarity of the drug [3]. Fat-soluble drugs penetrate the capillary wall more rapidly than water-soluble drugs [6]. In the extravascular space, pharmacons remain free in solution, bind to protein in interstitial fluid or attach to superficial coats of plasma cell membranes [3].

Only nonprotein-bound pharmacons enter the mammary alveolar or small duct cells. Most free pharmacons diffuse passively while others are actively transported through the basal lamina and plasma membrane. The plasma membrane consists of a lipid barrier with water-filled, protein-lined pores and, therefore, the rate of passage of a particular drug depends upon the degree of ionization and lipid solubility as well as the concentration gradient. Lipid-soluble, nonionized molecules pass freely through the plasma membrane whereas ionized pharmacons are transported by carrier proteins (ionophore transport) and water-soluble drugs of <200 molecular weight pass via the water-filled pores [5]. From the mammary cell pharmacons pass into milk either by apical pores (diffusion or active transport) or by merocrine or apocrine secretion. In milk, pharmacons are either free or bound to fat globules, to lipoproteins surrounding the globules or to protein granules. Binding may occur either prior to or after drug excretion from the cell [5].

Factors Influencing Drug Concentration in Milk

Most ingested drugs are excreted into milk despite the physiological filtration system. Normally most drugs are lower in concentration in milk than plasma and are present in undetectable or at least nontoxic levels in milk [7]. Seldom more than 1–2% of the maternal dose appears in milk. In the case of renal dysfunction, drugs may reach very high concentrations in milk. Some drugs which pass into milk in appreciable quantities are excreted as ineffective metabolites. For example, 50% of the antibiotic, chloramphenicol (chloromycetin) is excreted in this way. Other drugs, such as nicotine, may be metabolized by the infant [7]. Only a few drugs ingested by the mother are harmful to the breast-fed infant even when doses are excessive. However, some pharmacons administered at levels acceptable for adults may be toxic to infants due to the immaturity of hepatic and renal detoxification systems.

The concentration which a drug reaches in milk is dependent upon six major factors: drug dosage, proportion bound in plasma, molecular weight, lipid solubility, degree of ionization and pH difference between plasma and milk. Due to the controlled pH in plasma of 7.4, drugs which are weak acids are ionized to a greater extent and are protein-bound to a greater degree than weak alkaline drugs [3]. The distribution of a drug between plasma and milk can be estimated as a milk to plasma (M/P) concentration ratio by use of the Henderson-Hasselbalch equation [2] (fig. 2). Most drugs enter mammary alveolar cells in a nonionized, nonprotein-bound form. Under usual pH conditions, weak acidic drugs are less concentrated in milk than in plasma whereas weak alkaline drugs are more concentrated in milk. However, a decrease in plasma pH, as occurs in respiratory acidosis, would result in less ionization of an acidic drug and an increased M/P ratio. Some examples of weak acidic and alkaline drugs are shown in table I.

Table I. Classification of common drugs

Weak acids	Weak bases
Diuretics, methotrexate, nalidixic acid, phenobarbital, salicylate, streptomycin, sulfate, sulfonamide	alkaloids, amphetamines, antihistamines, caffeine, ephedrine, erythromycin, isoniazid, theophylline

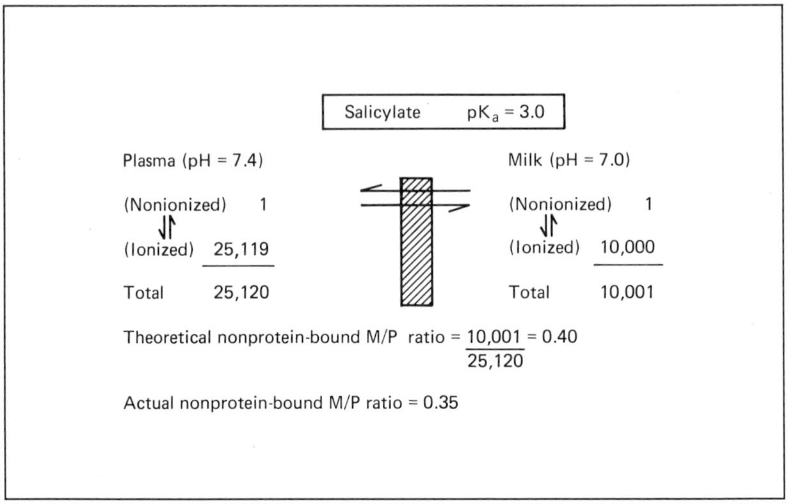

Fig. 2. Use of Henderson-Hasselbalch equation for theoretical determination of salicylate distribution across a semipermeable membrane between plasma and milk.

Selected Pharmacons and Their Risks to Breast-Fed Infants

Some categories of drugs contain pharmacons which should be limited or avoided by nursing mothers because of their potential harm to breast-fed infants; these are shown in table II. Among the pharmacons reported to be harmful to infants, some are based on extensive research, others on single case studies and still others are based on controversial evidence. Most studies have been done with single-dose or short-term drug administration; few data are available for continuous dosing or long-term drug administration. Measurements of drug concentration in milk as well as in blood, saliva, and urine of breast-fed infants are needed for more complete evaluation of the potential harm of a drug to infants. The drug categories to be discussed here were selected on the basis of their potential harm to the nursing infant. However, this is not intended to prejudice against the use of medications by lactating mothers.

Table II. Milk/plasma ratio of selected pharmacons and risks to the infant

Pharmacon	Use	Milk/plasma ratio	Possible effects on infant
Alkylating agents			
Ergot alkaloids	migraine		nausea, vomiting, diarrhea, weakness, unstable blood pressure
Methotrexate	tumors	0.10	none
Analgesics and anti-inflammatory			
Alphaprodine	pain		sedative effect
Acetaminophen	pain	low	hepatotoxicity
Antihistamines	inflammation bronchial constriction		maternal milk volume
Salicylates	pain, headache	0.05	impaired platelet function, kernicterus
Anti-coagulants			
Heparin (i.v.)	pain, headache	0	none
Metronidazole	pain, headache	0.6–1.4	prothrombin levels, hematoma
Phenindione	blood clotting prevention		postoperative hematoma, prolonged prothrombin and thromboplastin times
Warfarin	blood clotting prevention	0	none
Anticonvulsants			
Barbiturates	convulsions	low	hepatic microsomal enzyme activity, CNS depression
Phenobarbitone and phenytoin	convulsions, hyperactivity	0.17–0.28	methemoglobinemia, hepatic drug metabolizing enzymes
Anti-infective agents			
Ampicillin	infections		diarrhea
Chloramphenicol (Chloromycetin)	infections	0.5–0.6	anemia, bone marrow depression, vomiting
Metronidazole	vaginitis due to *Trichomonas vaginalis*	0.6–1.4	anorexia, vomiting, blood dyscrasia
Penicillin	infections	0.02–0.20	antigenic response
Sulfonamides		0.08–0.97	
Gantrisin	infections		neonatal jaundice, hemolytic anemia in G6PDH deficiency
Nalidixic acid	infections	0.08–0.13	hemolytic anemia
Nitrofurantoin	urinary tract infection		hemolytic anemia in G6PDH deficiency
Tetracycline	infections	0.63–0.8	none
CNS stimulants			
Methylxanthines	diuretic, headache,	0.8 (1.0)[a]	irritability
Caffeine	vasodilator, cardiac	0.7	
Theobromine	stimulant	0.8	
Theophylline			

[a] Percentage of maternal dose (theoretical) transmitted by human milk to the breast-fed infant.

Table II. (cont.)

Pharmacon	Use	Milk/plasma ratio	Possible effects on infant
Hormones			
Adrenaline	cardiac muscle depression		none
Corticotrophin (ACTH)	ketosis		none
Dihydrotachsterol (Hytakerol)	blood calcium regulator		hypercalcemia
Ethisterone (Pranone)	uterine bleeding	high	skeletal anomalies
Insulin	diabetes		none
Medroxyprogesterone acetate (Provera)	menstrual cycle anomalies	low	none
Naproxen	infections		hypoxemia, hypertension, kernicterus
Oral contraceptives	birth control		gynecomastia, vaginal proliferation, hyperbilirubinemia, maternal milk composition and volume altered
Laxatives			
Anthraquinone drugs	constipation		
Aloe, rhubarb		low	catharsis
Cascara, sagrada		high	catharsis
Senna		low	none
Colamel	constipation		catharsis
Phenolphthalein	constipation	low	catharsis
Minerals			
Iron	anemia	low	none
Provitamins			
Carotene			yellow discoloration of skin
Psychotherapeutic			
Choralhydrate (noctec, somnos)	inability to sleep	low	minimal sedation
Codeine	pain	2.0	addiction or prevention of withdrawal symptoms
Diazepam (Valium)	skeletal muscle tension	0.68	abnormal EEG, lethargy, weight loss, prolonged hyperbilirubinemia
Heroin	pain	low	addiction or prevention of withdrawal symptoms
Imipramine hydrochloride	depression	0.08–0.50	none
Lithium	manic-depressive disorders	0.35–0.36	hypotonia, cyanosis, muscle flaccidity, abnormal EEG
Morphine	pain	2.0	addiction or prevention of withdrawal symptoms
Tetrahydrocannabinol (Marijuana)			none
Thyroid affecting agents			
Carbimazole	hyperthyroidism	0.6	goiter
Iodide	goiter	3.0	goiter, agranulocytosis
Propylthiouracil	hyperthyroidism	low (0.77)[a]	none
Thiouracil	hyperthyroidism	3.0	goiter
Thyroxin	hypothyroidism	high	none

Table II. (cont.)

Pharmacon	Use	Milk/plasma ratio	Possible effects on infant
Vitamins			
Calciferol (vitamin D)	hypoparathyroidism	high	hypercalcemia
Cobalamin (vitamin B_{12})		low	none
Folic acid		0.23	none
Phytonadione (vitamin K)			↓ prothrombin time
Pyridoxine (vitamin B_6)	hyperkinesis, epilepsy, tardive dyskinesia, Parkinson's disease	0.1–0.25	
Thiamin (vitamin B_1)	beriberi treatment	high	none (in deficiency, excretion of toxic methylglyoxal may cause death)
Miscellaneous			
Alcohol		low	none (if moderate intake)
Antipyrine	study of hepatic drug metabolism	1.0	liver dysfunction
Chlorothiazide	diuretic	low	none
Fluorides	cavity prevention		mottling of teeth
Isoniazid	tuberculosis	1.0 (2.3)[a]	liver damage
Methadone	treatment of heroin addiction	0.3–0.83	death
Nicotine		low (0.17)[a]	no ill effect if mother smokes $\leq$ 20 cigarettes/day; > 20 causes vomiting, nausea, cramps, diarrhea, maternal secretion
Potassium iodide	cough preparation		goiter
Radioactive ^{131}I-iodine	lung scans	65.0	thyroid damage

[a] Percentage of maternal dose (theoretical) transmitted by human milk to the breast-fed infant.

Analgesics

Due largely to aspirin, analgesics are perhaps the most commonly used drugs during pregnancy and lactation [8]. In addition to aspirin, analgesics include phenacetin, acetaminophen and also psychotropic agents, such as codeine and morphine. Frequent use of analgesics during lactation has prompted, surprisingly, little research on the transport of these pharmacons into milk and their potential harm to the nursing infant. Present evidence suggests that aspirin may be the safest among available analgesics for nursing mothers.

Aspirin. Aspirin (acetylsalicylic acid) is an antipyretic and antiinflammatory agent as well as an analgesic [9]. These effects of the drug are produced by free salicylic acid and are dependent upon gastrointestinal hydrolysis of the acetyl derivative. The acetyl derivative of salicylic acid has been observed to dissociate bilirubin from serum albumin and prevent platelet aggregation [9] as well as to interfere with blood clotting [10]. However, salicylate, a weak acid, is highly ionized and extensively protein-bound in plasma and these properties limit its transport from plasma to milk. A maternal dose of 454 mg aspirin in pure form may reach a protein-bound M/P ratio of only 0.05 [11] whereas M/P ratios for higher doses are dependent upon saturation levels of the two major pathways for elimination of salicylate [9]. Unfortunately, saturation levels vary widely among individuals and an absolute limit cannot be established for lactating mothers [8]. Conservative administration of salicylate (60 mg/kg/day) results in a peak concentration of the drug in plasma around 1 h and plasma half-life at approximately 3 h [9]. Conservative doses of aspirin are not of concern; however, nursing mothers should avoid excessive use of aspirin since salicylate elimination in neonates may be restricted to one third that in adults [8].

Phenacetin, Acetaminophen, Morphine and Codeine. Both phenacetin and its major metabolite, acetaminophen (Tylenol), exert analgesic and antipyretic effects [12]. Similarly, morphine and its methyl derivative, codeine, are prescribed as analgesics. Hazards are greater in the use of the latter pharmacons by nursing mothers due to their addictive and basic ionic properties. Phenacetin and acetaminophen are hydrophilic, weakly acidic compounds which are transported only slightly into milk [11]. Accurate M/P ratios for these drugs are not available since in the single study of their transfer into milk, the compounds were given simultaneously and phenacetin is known to readily metabolize to acetaminophen [11]. Data suggest that acetaminophen, whether administered directly or synthesized from phenacetin, is cleared more slowly by the infant than the adult. For this reason, large doses of phenacetin or acetaminophen are not advisable for nursing mothers.

Codeine is metabolized to morphine [12] and its pharmacologic properties are dependent solely upon this conversion. Both codeine and morphine are transported readily into milk [11]; the lower protein binding capacity of codeine results in a slightly greater transfer of this drug into milk compared to morphine [13]. Both pharmacons are weakly basic and lipophilic in nature and may show high M/P ratios, ≥2.0 [11]. Despite some metabolic inactivation of morphine and codeine by the mother and infant, the use of these analgesics by nursing mothers is contraindicated. Analgesics should be selected with caution for the well-being of the breast-fed infant.

Central Nervous System Stimulants

Caffeine, Theophylline and Theobromine. Caffeine (1,3,7-trimethyl xanthine) and similarly structured theophylline (1,3-dimethyl xanthine) and theobromine (3,7-dimethyl xanthine) are central nervous system stimulants and bronchial dilators [14]. Their presence in many beverages and foods (caffeine and theobromine in coffee, tea and chocolate) increases the likelihood of methyl xanthine ingestion by lactating mothers. Therapeutic use of methyl xanthines (caffeine, in particular) should be limited in nursing mothers due to the relative ease of transport of the drugs across plasma-milk barriers and the restricted clearance of these compounds by the newborn. Caffeine and theophylline rapidly penetrate the capillary wall and membranes of the mammary glandular cell to reach high M/P ratios [11]. An average nonprotein-bound M/P ratio for caffeine has been reported to be 0.82 [11] and for theophylline approximately 0.73 [15]. However, the percent of an oral dose which appears in milk is dependent upon the extent of protein binding in plasma. Theophylline is more extensively bound (50%) than caffeine (25%) and, consequently, only 10% of an oral dose of theophylline is found in milk [15, 16] whereas 66% of a caffeine dose may be excreted into milk [11]. Both caffeine and theophylline require remarkably long clearance times in the newborn [11]. Although elimination pathways are the same as for adults, caffeine half-times in plasma of infants are nearly 17-fold those of adults [17, 18]. Similarly, theophylline clearance in the infant is many times slower than in the adult [15]. Theophylline and caffeine should be consumed in moderation by nursing mothers. Although reports of caffeine and theophylline toxicity in infants are restricted to direct administration [19] or to uncontrolled and controversial case studies, nursing mothers are advised to wait until after the peak in methyl xanthines in plasma (0.5–1 h) before breast-feeding [15]. In contrast to theophylline and caffeine, theobromine has weak pharmacologic properties and is not a therapeutic agent [1]. Although it has an average M/P ratio of 0.82 and a plasma half-life of 9.8 h [20], the quantity in food is so small that even chocolate restriction during lactation is unwarranted [1].

Psychotherapeutic Agents

Psychotherapeutic agents are used widely by nursing mothers [21] but, unfortunately, studies of the transport of individual agents into milk are limited and are not quantitative [22]. Information is incomplete regarding the transport of thioxanthenes (antidepressants), tricyclic antidepressants, phenothiazines (tranquilizers) and monoamine oxidase inhibitors (antidepressants) into human milk. Some drugs, such as the antiemetic haloperidol, are considered safe for use by nursing mothers solely on the basis of their widespread use and no reports of adverse effects [23]. Three psychotherapeutic agents for which considerable data exist are diazepam, tetrahydrocannabinol (THC) and lithium carbonate. Evidence suggests that use of diazepam and lithium carbonate during lactation presents some hazards to the breast-fed infant whereas the effects of THC are not completely known.

Diazepam. The tranquilizer diazepam (Valium) is one of the most commonly prescribed psychotherapeutic agents in the world [22]. It is administered often during pregnancy and lactation to relieve anxiety and tension [24]. During metabolism, diazepam is demethylated and hydroxylated to yield oxazepam, a metabolite which also possesses tranquilizer activity [22]. The first evidence of diazepam transfer into milk was reported by *Patrick* et al. [25], who observed lethargy, weight loss and an EEG compatible with sedation in the breast-fed infant of a mother administered 30 mg/diazepam/day. Also, oxazepam was observed in the infant's urine. *Erkkola and Kanto* [24] administered a similar dose of 30 mg diazepam/day to 3 lactating women for 6 days and observed an M/P ratio of 0.10 for combined diazepam and its demethylated form at 4 days and 0.12 after 6 days of treatment but no oxazepam was found in milk. Diazepam levels in milk increased consistently over the treatment period whereas diazepam and demethylated diazepam decreased significantly in the serum of the infant during the last 2 days of the 6-day period of breast-feeding, suggesting maturation of the elimination pathway for diazepam in the infants [24]. Diazepam is detoxified by conjugation with glucuronic acid, the same mechanism as for bilirubin excretion. Hence, *Ayd* [22] warns that competition for glucuronic acid by diazepam may result in hyperbilirubinemia and possibly kernicterus in breast-fed infants of Valium-treated mothers [26]. Both *Patrick* et al. [25] and *Erkkola and Kanto* [24] advise that mothers receiving diazepam should not breast-feed.

Tetrahydrocannabinol. Marijuana, derived from the hemp plant, *Cannabis sativa,* is one of the most widely used illicit drugs [26]. Δ-9-Tetrahydrocannabinol (Δ9-THC) is considered the most potent psychoactive component of marijuana [27]; however, its 11-hydroxy-metabolite that forms in human liver appears to have even higher pharmacologic activity [26]. As much as 90–95% of an oral dose of Δ9-THC may be absorbed from the gastrointestinal tract [26], and this is strongly bound to plasma lipoproteins [28]. Therefore, only small quantities of the drug are reported to be transferred into milk of laboratory animals [29]. The percent of an oral dose which appears in milk in 4 h is approximately 0.02 [29] and only 0.2% is reported to pass into milk in a 24-hour collection [30]. Excretion of Δ9-THC into milk of laboratory animals is low; however, similar low levels of excretion into human milk cannot be assumed. This pharmacon is known to induce symptoms of conjunctiva congestion, increased heart rate [28], hypertension and severe headache in man [27]. Since the half-life of Δ9-THC in plasma in man may be as long as two days, nursing mothers should be cautious in the use of this pharmacon until further research is done [31].

Lithium. Presently lithium carbonate is used principally in the treatment of the manic phase of manic-depressive disorders [32]. The well-being of breast-fed infants may be jeopardized by mothers who ingest lithium since its toxicity is well documented [33]. Also, the drug is possibly teratogenic [34, 35] and goitrogenic [36]. The M/P ratio of lithium is approximately 0.5 and shows little variance over time [22, 37]. This high ratio suggests that the breast-fed infant ingests potentially harmful amounts of lithium from the mother's dose [38]. *Wilbanks* et al. [39] presented the first report of lithium toxicity in the newborn of a lithium-treated mother. Symptoms of cyanosis, hypotonia and an abnormal EEG pattern were observed and these were reported also for the infant of another lithium-treated mother [32]. A third case of lithium toxicity was noted in the newborn of a mother accustomed to a daily oral dose of 600–1,200 mg lithium [38]. The toxic symptoms, noted at birth, recurred when the mother initiated breast-feeding and these persisted until nursing was discontinued. Because lithium levels in milk may be less than that to which the infant was exposed in utero (lithium completely crosses the placental barrier), some physicians argue that lithium-treated mothers can safely breast-feed [35]. However, symptoms of lithium toxicity in the newborn are prolonged by breast-feeding [38] and bottle feeding is recommended for lithium-treated mothers [32].

Antibiotics and Chemotherapeutic Agents

Antibiotics include a wide range of pharmacons which show highly variable degrees of transfer into human milk. Although most antibiotics administered to nursing mothers are considered safe for the breast-fed infant [40], several antibacterial agents have been implicated in health complications of the newborn. Unfortunately, evidence supporting the hazards of these drugs are often single case studies and, for this reason, the data are far from conclusive.

Sulfonamides include three pharmacons that may be harmful to breast-fed infants. Nalidixic acid has been suggested to cause hemolytic anemia in normal infants [23] and nitrofurantoin and sulfamethoxypyridazine (Gantrisin) to provoke kernicterus as well as hemolytic anemia in glucose-6-phosphate-deficient infants [7]. Apart from the sulfonamides, various anti-infective agents, including chloramphenicol, metronidazole and ampicillin, are considered potentially harmful pharmacons for mothers who breast-feed. Chloramphenicol and metronidazole have been implicated in a number of health problems in nursing infants. Chloramphenicol may cause anemia, bone marrow depression and vomiting in the nursing infant [7]; metronidazole has been implicated in infantile anorexia, vomiting and blood dyscragia [2]. Maternal administration of ampicillin may result in diarrhea in the breast-fed infant. Maternal intake of the chemotherapeutic agent isoniazid is contraindicated. The drug is acetylated in the liver to a toxic form which may result in infantile hepatic toxicity [1]. Data are scarce on the harmful effects of antibiotic ingestion by nursing mothers; however, these drugs should be prescribed only in moderate dosages to nursing mothers and the length of administration should be limited [40]. Prolonged ingestion of antibacterial agents by nursing mothers may ultimately precipitate alterations in the intestinal flora of the breast-fed infant and this in turn could effect the immune defense mechanism of the infant [40].

Oral Contraceptives. Oral contraceptives (OC) are commonly prescribed at 6 weeks postpartum [41] to protect the puerpera from pregnancy [42], to aid in uterus involution and to initiate the return of menses [43]. These drugs alter levels of several nutrients in plasma [44], reduce milk production [45], and may enter milk in appreciable quantities [46]. These changes are influenced by the type, quantity, and length of OC use [47]. The estrogen component (commonly, ethinyl estradiol and/or mestranol) appears to be responsible primarily for the alterations [47].

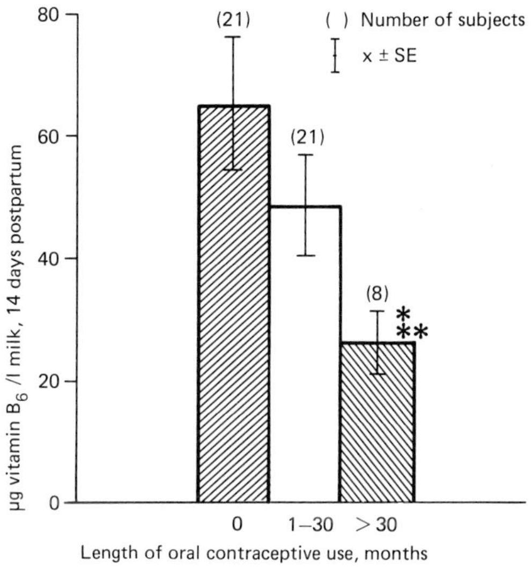

Fig. 3. Vitamin B_6 content in milk at 14 days postpartum in relation to months of oral contraceptive (OC) use. * Different ($p < 0.02$) from 1 to 30 months OC use. ** Different ($p < 0.003$) from no OC use.

Levels of vitamin B_6 have been observed to be significantly lower in plasma and milk of long-term OC users compared to levels for nonusers [48, 49]. Thus, qualitative changes in human milk as well as reduction in milk volume, precipitated by OC use, may endanger the well-being of breast-fed infants. In our laboratory, *Roepke and Kirksey* [48] noted that mothers of infants with unsatisfactory Apgar scores had low levels of vitamin B_6 in their serum and milk. At 14 days postpartum, vitamin B_6 in milk was only 26 µg/l for long-term OC users (> 30 months) or approximately one half that of nonusers (fig. 3). The ratio of vitamin B_6/protein in milk also was significantly lower for OC users compared to nonusers and the adequacy of vitamin B_6 was questioned especially relative to the protein content in milk of long-term OC users. Also in this laboratory, *West and Kirksey* [49] observed that the mother of a breast-fed infant, who suffered milk periodic seizures the first weeks of life, had a low vitamin B_6 intake (1.5 mg/day). Analysis of the mother's milk showed that it contained only

Table III. Levels of vitamin B_6 in biological fluids of a mother and her breast-fed infant who showed symptoms of a central nervous system disorder at 7 days of age

5 months gestation[1]		Delivery	Postpartum		
			7 days[2]	17 days	6 weeks
Mother[3]		PLP, ng/ml			
Plasma	24.9	3.4	–	35.5	51.0
		vitamin B_6, µg/l			
Milk	–	–	16	204	255
Infant		PLP, ng/ml			
Plasma	–	20.3[4]	2.8	51.5	–

[1] Mother supplemented with 5 mg pyridoxine · HCl/day from 3 months gestation.
[2] Mother's supplement changed from 5 to 20 mg pyridoxine · HCl/day.
[3] Used oral contraceptives for 10 years prior to pregnancy.
[4] Cord plasma.

67 µg vitamin B_6/l at 1 month postpartum. Her infant became asymptomatic after the introduction of cereal which contained 20–60 mg vitamin B_6. We postulated that the mother's low intake of vitamin B_6 in conjunction with low tissue reserves following long-term (3.5 years) use of OC resulted in poor maternal vitamin B_6 nutriture which was reflected in inadequate vitamin B_6 in her milk for the infant.

Recently, *Kirksey and Roepke* [50] determined levels of vitamin B_6 in the biological fluids of a 36-year-old primigravida and her breast-fed infant who developed symptoms of a CNS disorder at 7 days of age (table III). The symptoms included hyperactivity, shrill cries and rigid opisthotonos with transient cyanosis in the absence of other signs of illness. The mother had used OC for 10 years prior to pregnancy and had discontinued the use for only a few weeks prior to conception. At delivery, vitamin B_6 levels in maternal and cord plasma were approximately one half the expected levels and, at 7 days postpartum, vitamin B_6 content in milk was very low. Also at this time, the level of pyridoxal phosphate in plasma of the infant was extremely low and neurological symptoms were evident. The mother's pyridoxine supplement was increased immediately from 5 to 20 mg/day resulting in a marked increase in vitamin B_6 in milk. Subsequently the infant became asymptomatic without medication. At 17 days postpartum, vitamin B_6 parameters of the mother and infant were improved markedly.

Transfer of OC into human milk provides additional hazards to the breast-fed infant. *Curtis* [51] noted breast enlargement in a male infant shortly after maternal administration of mestranol (2.5 mg Enovid/day) and a return to normal size 2–3 weeks after breast-feeding was discontinued. The extent to which a specific sex hormone enters human milk depends upon the extent of its binding to serum globulins [46]. Testosterone preparations, such as norgestrel and norethisterone, show high affinities to sex hormone-binding-globulins and, therefore, little transfer into milk (M/P ratios of about 0.15). Progestins vary widely in their affinities to serum globulins but may show M/P ratios as high as 0.8 [46]. Mestranol and estradiol are assumed to have low binding capacities in plasma and therefore potentially high transfer into milk [42]. Because these estrogens are commonly included in OC preparations nursing mothers are advised to refrain from taking OC until breast-feeding is well established [44].

Vitamin B_6

The influence of pharmacologic doses of vitamin B_6 (pyridoxine) on lactation had been a source of controversy for the last 10 years. Megadoses of this vitamin are employed not only to treat conditions such as hyperkinesis [52], certain forms of epilepsy [53], tardive dyskinesia [54] and Parkinson's disease [55] but also to alleviate vitamin B_6 deficiencies and to prevent antagonistic deficiencies that accompany the administration of hydrazide-type drugs.

Although pyridoxine passes freely from plasma into milk, the controversy about megadoses concerns quantitative rather than qualitative influences of pyridoxine on milk. *Foukas* [56] first proposed that pyridoxine was an effective lactation inhibitor. Studies by *Marcus* [57] and *McIntosh* [58] confirmed that 600 mg vitamin B_6/day suppressed lactation and lowered prolactin levels [57]. *Delitala* et al. [59] confirmed *McIntosh's* [58] finding and further noted that vitamin B_6 elevated growth hormone levels. Megadoses of pyridoxine were proposed to increase the conversion of dopa to dopamine [59] which either inhibited prolactin or released its inhibitor [60].

Most recent human studies [61–63] fail to confirm the findings of earlier studies and suggest that megadoses of vitamin B_6 have no effect on lactation, prolactin or growth hormone levels. Decarboxylase which converts dopa to dopamine also converts 5-hydroxytryptophan to serotonin and therefore the lack of effect of pyridoxine on prolactin levels may be due to the simultaneous stimulation of both dopaminergic and serotonergic activities. Also the quantity of pyridoxine in maternal supplements (1–20 mg) is less than 1/30th the levels used in studies of lactation inhibition. Findings from our laboratory [64] show that 20 mg pyridoxine·HCl/day did not significantly effect the milk volume of nursing mothers.

Precautions in Drug Use by Nursing Mothers

Only a few drugs are contraindicated for nursing mothers; however, the following precautions may minimize the risks of some potentially harmful pharmacons to breast-fed infants: (1) All unnecessary medications should be avoided by nursing mothers. (2) If medications are necessary during lactation, drug dosage should be well-controlled and the infant monitored closely for any adverse symptoms. (3) Drugs should be administered shortly after breast-feeding and the interval prolonged before the next feeding in order to minimize the infant's exposure to the pharmacon. (4) If the infant must be fed soon after a potentially harmful drug has been administered to the mother, bottle-feeding is recommended.

References

1 Berlin, C.M.: Pharmacologic considerations of drug use in the lactating mother. Obstet. Gynec., N.Y. *58:* 175–235 (1981).

2 Berlin, C.M.: The excretion of drugs in human milk; in Drug and chemical risks to the fetus and newborn, pp. 115–127 (Liss, New York 1979).

3 Vorherr, H.: The breast: morphology, physiology and lactation (Academic Press, New York 1974).

4 O'Brien, T.: Excretion of drugs in human milk. Am. J. Hosp. Pharm. *31:* 844–854 (1974).

5 Berlin, C.M.: The excretion of drugs in human milk. Prog. clin. biol. Res. *36:* 115–127 (1980).

6 Schanker, L.S.: Passage of drugs across body membranes. Pharmac. Rev. *14:* 501–521 (1962).

7 Platzher, A.C.D.; Lew, C.D.; Stewart, D.: Drug administration via breastmilk. Hosp. Pract. *1980:* 111–122.

8 Levy, G.; Garrettson, J.K.: Kinetics of salicylate elimination by newborn infants of mothers who ingested aspirin before delivery. Pediatrics, Springfield *53:* 201–220 (1974).

9 Levy, G.: Clinical pharmacokinetics of aspirin. Pediatrics, Springfield *62:* 867–872 (1978).

10 Corby, D.G.; Shulman, I.: The effects of antenatal drug administration on aggregation of newborn infants. J. Pediat. *79:* 307 (1971).
11 Findlay, J.W.A.; Deangelis, R.L.; Kearney, M.F.; Welch, R.M.; Findlay, J.M.: Analgesic drugs in breastmilk and plasma. Clin. Pharmacol. Ther. *29:* 625–633 (1981).
12 Findlay, J.W.A.; Jones, E.C.; Butz, R.F.; Welch, R.M.: Plasma codeine and morphine concentrations after therapeutic oral doses of codeine containing analgesics. Clin. Pharmacol. Ther. *24:* 60–68 (1978).
13 Baggot, J.D.; Davis, L.E.: Species differences in plasma protein binding of morphine and codeine. Am. J. vet. Res. *34:* 571–574 (1973).
14 Aranda, J.V.; Cook, C.E.; Gorman, W.; Collinge, J.M.; Loughnan, P.M.; Buterbridge, E.W.; Aldridge, A.; Neims, A.H.: Pharmacokinetic profile of caffeine in the newborn infant with apnea. J. Pediat. *94:* 663–668 (1979).
15 Yurchak, A.M.; Jusko, W.J.: Theophylline secretion into breastmilk. Pediatrics, Springfield *57:* 518–520 (1976).
16 Stec, G.P.; Greenberger, P.; Ruo, T.I.; Henthorn, T.; Morita, Y.; Atkinson, A.J.; Patterson, R.: Kinetics of theophylline transfer to breastmilk. Clin. Pharmacol. Ther. *28:* 404–408 (1980).
17 Marks, V.; Kelley, J.F.: Absorption of caffeine from tea, coffee and coca cola. Lancet *i:* 827 (1973).
18 Gorodescher, R.; Karplus, M.; Worsjawski, D.; Bark, H.; Moses, S.W.; Gorden, C.: Caffeine pharmacokinetics in the neonate: human and animal studies. Pediat. Res. *11:* 1013 (1977).
19 Brem, A.S.; Martin, H.; Stern, L.: Toxicity from tea ingestion in an infant: a computer simulation analysis. Clin. Biochem. *10:* 148–150 (1977).
20 Resman, B.H.; Blumenthal, H.P.; Jusko, W.J.: Breastmilk distribution of theobromine from chocolate. J. Pediat. *91:* 477–480 (1977).
21 Wilson, J.T.; Brown, R.D.; Cherek, D.R.; Barley, J.W.; Hilman, B.; Jobe, P.C.; Manno, B.R.; Manno, J.E.; Redetzki, H.M.; Stewart, J.J.: Drug excretion in human breastmilk: principles, pharmacokinetics and projected consequences. Clin. Pharmacokinet. *5:* 1–66 (1980).
22 Ayd, F.J.: Excretion of psychotropic drugs in human breastmilk. Int. Drug Ther. Newsl. *8:* 33 (1973).
23 Berley, L.: Drugs and breast-feeding. Clin. Obstet. Gynec. *8:* 291–295 (1981).
24 Erkkola, R.; Kanto, J.: Diazepam and breast-feeding. Lancet *i:* 1235–1236 (1972).
25 Patrick, M.J.; Tilstone, W.J.; Reavey, P.: Diazepam and breast-feeding. Lancet *i:* 543–544 (1972).
26 Lemberger, L.; Ruben, A.: The physiologic disposition of marijuana in man. Life Sci. *17:* 1637–1642 (1976).
27 Hosko, M.J.; Kochar, M.S.; Wang, R.I.H.: Effects of orally administered delta-9-tetrahydrocannabinol in man. Clin. Pharmacol. Ther. *14:* 344–351 (1972).
28 Perez-Reyes, M.; Lipton, M.A.; Timmons, M.C.; Wall, M.E.; Brine, D.R.; Davis, K.H.: Pharmacology of orally administered Δ^9-tetrahydrocannabinol. Clin. Pharmacol. Ther. *14:* 48–55 (1972).
29 Jakuboric, A.; Tait, R.M.; McGreer, P.L.: Excretion of THC and its metabolites in ewe's milk. Toxicol. appl. Pharmacol. *28:* 38–43 (1974).
30 Chao, F.; Green, D.E.; Forrest, I.S.; Kaplan, J.W.; Winship-Ball, A.; Braude, M.: The

passage of ^{14}C-Δ-9-tetrahydrocannabinol into the milk of lactating squirrel monkeys. Res. Commun. chem. Pathol. Pharmacol. *15:* 303–317 (1976).
31 Ohlsson, A.; Lindgren, J.E.; Wahlen, A.; Agurell, S.; Hollister, L.E.; Gillespie, H.K.: Plasma delta-9-tetrahydrocannabinol concentrations and clinical effects after oral and intravenous administration and smoking. Clin. Pharmacol. Ther. *28:* 409–415 (1980).
32 Woody, J.W.; London, W.L.; Wilbanks, G.D.: Lithium toxicity in a newborn. Pediatrics, Springfield *47:* 94–96 (1971).
33 Corcoran, A.C.; Taylor, R.D.; Page, L.H.: Lithium poisoning from the use of salt substitutes. J. Am. med. Ass. *138:* 685 (1949).
34 Vacaflor, L.; Lehmann, H.E.; Ban, T.A.: Side effects and teratogenicity of lithium carbonate treatment. Clin. Pharmacol. Ther. *10:* 387–389 (1970).
35 Fries, J.: Lithium in pregnancy. Lancet *i:* 1233 (1970).
36 Berens, S.C.; Wolff, J.; Murray, A.L.: Lithium concentration by the thyroid. Endocrinology *87:* 1085–1096 (1970).
37 Schou, M.; Amdisen, A.: Lithium and pregnancy. III. Lithium ingestion by children breast-fed by women on lithium treatment. Br. med. J. *ii:* 138 (1973).
38 Tunnesson, W.W.; Hertz, C.G.: Toxic effects of lithium in new born infants: a commentary. Pediatrics, Springfield *81:* 804–807 (1972).
39 Wilbanks, G.D.; Bressler, B.; Peite, C.H.; Cherng, W.B.; London, W.L.: Toxic effects of lithium carbonate in a mother and newborn infant. J. Am. med. Ass. *213:* 865–867 (1970).
40 Rivera-Calimlin, L.: Drugs in breastmilk. Drug Ther. *7:* 59–63 (1977).
41 Karim, M.; Ammar, R.; Elmahgoub, S.; Elganzoury, B.; Fikri, F.; Abdou, I.: Injected progestogen and lactation. Br. med. J. *i:* 200–203 (1971).
42 Schwallie, P.C.: The effect of depot-medroxy progesterone acetate on the fetus and nursing infant. A review. Contraception *23:* 375–386 (1981).
43 Gantrell, R.D.: Immediate postpartum contraception. Obstet. Gynec., N.Y. *36:* 101–106 (1970).
44 Lonnerdahl, B.; Forsum, E.; Hambraeus, L.: Effect of oral contraceptives on composition and volume of breastmilk. Am. J. clin. Nutr. *33:* 816–824 (1980).
45 Kader, M.M.A.; Hay, A.A.; El-Safouri, S.; Aziz, M.T.A.; El-Din, J.S.; Kamal, I.; Hefnawi, F.; Ghoneim, M.; Talaat, M.; Younis, N.; Tagui, A.; Abdalla, M.: Clinical, biochemical and experimental studies on lactation. III. Biochemical changes induced in human milk by gestagens. Am. J. Obstet. Gynec. *105:* 978–984 (1969).
46 Nilsson, S.; Nygren, K.G.; Johansson, E.D.B.: *D*-Norgestrel concentrations in maternal plasma, milk and child plasma during administration of oral contraceptives to nursing women. Am. J. Obstet. Gynec. *129:* 178–184 (1977).
47 Cumming, F.J.: Effect of oral contraceptives use on ascorbic acid and vitamin A in lactation. J. hum. Nutr., Lond. *35:* 249–256 (1981).
48 Roepke, J.L.B.; Kirksey, A.: Vitamin B_6 nutriture during pregnancy and lactation. II. The effect of long-term use of oral contraceptives. Am. J. clin. Nutr. *32:* 2257–2264 (1979).
49 West, K.D.; Kirksey, A.: Influence of vitamin B_6 intake on the content of the vitamin in human milk. Am. J. clin. Nutr. *29:* 961–969 (1976).
50 Kirksey, A.; Roepke, J.L.B.: Vitamin B_6 nutriture of mothers of three breast-fed deonates with central nervous system disorders. Fed. Proc. *40:* 3602 (1981).

51 Curtis, E.M.: Oral contraceptive feminization of a normal male infant. Obstet. Gynec., N.Y. *23:* 295 (1964).
52 Coleman, M.; Steinberg, G.; Tippett, J.; Bhagavan, H.M.; Coursin, D.B.; Gross, M.; Lewis, C.; Deveau, L.: A preliminary study of the effect of pyridoxine administration in a subgroup of hyperkinetic children: a double-blind crossover comparison with methylphenidate. Biol. Psychiat. *14:* 741–751 (1979).
53 Lott, F.T.; Coulombe, B.A.; Dipaolo, R.V.; Richardson, E.P.; Levy, H.L.: Vitamin B_6-dependent seizures: pathology and chemical findings in brain. Neurology, Minneap. *24:* 47–54 (1978).
54 Deveaugh, J.; Geiss, M.D.; Laurenie Manion, A.B.: High dose pyridoxine in tardive dyskinesia. J. clin. Psychiat. *39:* 573–575 (1978).
55 Holtz, P.; Palm, D.: Pharmacological aspects of vitamin B_6. Pharmac. Rev. *16:* 113–178 (1964).
56 Foukas, M.D.: An antilactogenic effect of pyridoxine. J. Obstet. Gynec. *80:* 718–720 (1973).
57 Marcus, R.G.: Suppression of lactation with high doses of pyridoxine. S. Afr. med. J. *6:* 2155–2156 (1975).
58 McIntosh, E.N.: Treatment of women with galactorrhea-amenorrhea syndrome with pyridoxine (vit. B_6). J. clin. Endocr. Metab. *42:* 1192–1195 (1976).
59 Delitala, G.; Masala, A.; Alagna, S.; Devilla, L.: Effect of pyridoxine in human hypophysealtrophic hormone release: possible stimulation of hypothalamic dopaminergic pathway. J. clin. Endocr. Metab. *42:* 603–606 (1976).
60 Kochenour, N.K.; Emery, M.G.: Drugs in lactating women. Obstet. Gynec. Annu. *10:* 107–126 (1982).
61 Tolis, G.; Laliberte, R.; Guyda, H.; Naftolin, F.: Ineffectiveness of pyridoxine (B_6) to alter secretion of growth hormone and prolactin and absence of therapeutic effects on galactorrhea-amenorrhea syndrome. J. clin. Endocr. Metab. *44:* 1197–1199 (1977).
62 Lehtovirta, P.; Ranta, T.; Seppala, M.: Pyridoxine treatment of galactorrhea-amenorrhea syndromes. Acta endocrin., Copenh. *87:* 682–686 (1978).
63 Goodenow, T.J.; Malarky, W.B.: Ineffectiveness of pyridoxine in evaluation and treatment of hyperprolactinemic amenorrhea-galactorrhea syndrome. Am. J. Obstet. Gynec. *133:* 161–164 (1979).
64 Styslinger, L.M.; Kirksey, A.: Effects of different levels of vitamin B_6 supplementation during lactation on vitamin B_6 content in milk and vitamin B_6 intakes of breast-fed infants. Fed. Proc. *41:* 1188 (1982).

A. Kirksey, PhD, Department of Food and Nutrition, Purdue University,
West Lafayette, IN 47907 (USA)

Wld Rev. Nutr. Diet., vol. 43, pp. 80–94 (Karger, Basel 1984)

Food, Formula and Drug Effects on the Disposition of Nutrients

Daphne A. Roe

Division of Nutritional Sciences, Cornell University, Ithaca, N.Y., USA

Past definition and separation of nutrients and drugs by usage, vehicle and disposition are no longer tenable. Previously nutrients were exclusively contained in foods and drugs were largely contained in medications. Vitamins are now consumed in the form of pills, capsules, pediatric formulas, defined chemical diets, health foods and enriched foods as well as in natural food sources. Total daily intakes may greatly exceed the physiological requirements. Despite the fact that vitamins are often ingested as mixtures, with or without food and often with medications, dietary and drug factors which influence the bioavailability of these pharmacological doses of vitamins have not recently been reviewed.

Diet-related factors and drugs which affect the bioavailability of pharmacological doses of vitamins or vitamins taken in pharmaceutical formulation can be broadly subdivided into those which are related to direct vitamin-food interactions or vitamin-drug interactions, and those which are related to effects of food or drugs on gastrointestinal function. A classification, based on this subdivision, which is applicable to diet and drug factors affecting vitamin uptake is shown in table I. In order to adapt this classification to practical use, it is necessary both to identify diet components and drugs which alter the bioavailability of specific fat and water-soluble vitamins and to show the net outcome of concurrent intake. Specific goals are (1) to develop an operational framework which will allow prediction of relative vitamin bioavailability when the form, formulation vehicle, diet and drugs are known, and (2) to examine parallels between effect of food on vitamin and drug bioavailability.

Table I. Physicochemical and functional characteristics of diet and drugs which affect vitamin bioavailability

	Diet	Drugs
Physicochemical characteristics		
Formulation	solid, liquid, natural food, fortification, semisynthetics, synthetic	liquid, suspension tablets, capsules, enteric coating, micronization
Components	proteins, amino acids, carbohydrate, fat, fiber, additives, alcohol	active drug, diluent, coating
Processing, preparation and storage	mode of preservation, cooking, light exposure	manufacture, mixture, shelf life
Physical factors	bulk, viscosity, osmolality, temperature, fluid volume	dissociation constant, lipid solubility, dissolution, particle size, ion exchange, adsorption, complexation
Functional characteristics		
Stomach emptying rate	decreased rate with solid, hot meals or high osmolality; increased rate with high fluid intake	decreased rate with anticholinergics
Intestinal motility	increased	increased with laxatives
Splanchnic blood flow	increased	increased cardiovascular drugs
GI secretion	increased	decreased with H_2 receptor antagonists
Active absorption	increased	competitive or decreased with antagonist
GI metabolism	change with dietary protein or carbohydrate	suppression with antibiotics

Model Vitamins

In order to study food variables which alter the bioavailability of pharmacological agents, model drugs are selected for animal and human investigations. Criteria for selection of these model drugs include well-characterized pharmacokinetic parameters, representativeness and low toxicity. Only some of the same criteria can be used in the selection of model vitamins. In the present context model vitamins have been selected to develop our conceptual framework because their absorption and gastrointestinal metabolism is well known, because the diet-related and drug factors which affect their bioavailability represent the known range of such factors. Thus, retinol and the provitamin, β-carotene, have been chosen as model fat-soluble vitamins and riboflavin has been selected as an example of a model water-soluble vitamin.

β-Carotene and Vitamin A: Sources, Site and Mechanism of Absorption

Dietary Factors Affecting Bioavailability

β-Carotene, being a hydrocarbon, is best absorbed when it is in an oily solution. Dietary fat promotes absorption and, as shown by *Roels* et al. [29], a small fat supplement added to a low fat diet enhances the absorption of this vitamin. Absorption of β-carotene from the aqueous environment of the small intestine requires that the vitamin be in micellar solution. Formation of micelles is promoted by release of bile and hence of bile salts into the gut lumen which in turn is stimulated by fat [9]. Lecithin has been reported to promote carotene absorption. *Wolf* [36] indicates that the lecithin effect is probably due to the non-specific effect of this phospholipid on micelle formation.

Conversion of β-carotene to retinol occurs in the intestinal mucosal cells. The enzyme which cleaves the β-carotene molecule is a dioxygenase (15-15′-dioxygenase) which is present in the cytosol. For activity of the dioxygenase, the presence of molecular oxygen and Fe^{++} are required but for maximal activity glutathione, bile salts, α-tocopherol and lecithin are also required. The initial product of cleavage of β-carotene is retinal and the retinal is then reduced to retinol by alcohol dehydrogenase which is also present as a mucosal enzyme. It is suggested that the α-tocopherol functions to prevent non-enzymatic oxidation of β-carotene or retinol [36]. Effects of α-tocopherol on the bioavailability of β-carotene depend on the amount present and on whether it is present in the intestine concurrently with the β-carotene during the absorption process. Although α-tocopherol in physiological amounts promotes β-carotene conversion to retinol, in excess α-tocopherol interferes with the accessibility of β-carotene to the mucosal dioxygenase enzyme [1].

The activity of the intestinal dioxygenase enzyme is increased by dietary protein. *Stoecker and Arnrich* [32] demonstrated that a high protein meal has an immediate effect on the conversion of β-carotene to retinal. The amount of β-carotene converted to retinal is limited by the capacity of the dioxygenase enzyme [11]. The dioxygenase enzyme occurs in the liver as well as in the intestine but, when carotene is administered by mouth, cleavage by the intestinal enzyme is much more active than by the liver enzyme and therefore the intestinal dioxygenase is more nutritionally important [37].

In a rat study conducted by *Gronowska-Senger* et al. [12], it was shown that utilization of β-carotene was promoted by inclusion of 5% fiber in the diet. The fiber consisted in a mixture of methyl cellulose, agar, wheat grain and pectin in equal parts. When more fiber was added to the rat diets, utilization of β-carotene decreased and more of the vitamin appeared in the feces. The authors concluded that while fiber is necessary for optimum utilization of β-carotene, a dietary fiber content of more than 10% had a negative effect on absorption of this vitamin. These findings may possibly indicate an effect of change in intestinal transit time on carotene absorption. However, presently the mechanism responsible for this fiber effect in rats is unclear and the relevance of these observations to human subjects is unknown.

Barnard and Heaton [3] found that large doses of another fiber source, lignin, had no effect on serum vitamin A values after an oral load. This finding was interpreted to mean that lignin had no effect on absorption of the vitamin. It has been proposed that lignin could reduce vitamin A absorption by interference with the micellar phase or by direct hydrophobic interaction with the vitamin [4].

When vitamin A is ingested in the form of retinyl esters, the esters are hydrolyzed by a hydrolase in the intestinal lumen and by a hydrolysate in the brush border. Free retinol is then transported into the intestinal mucosal cells when the retinol is again esterified by mucosal esterases. As with β-carotene, bile salts and α-tocopherol are also required for optimal retinol absorption. Autooxidation of dietary polyunsaturated fatty acids can cause destruction of retinol unless α-tocopherol is present. Dietary protein also promotes retinol absorption, though it is not known whether this protein effect is immediate or delayed [30]. Diet-related factors which influence the absorption of β-carotene and retinol are shown in figures 1 and 2.

Drug-Induced Malabsorption of β-Carotene and Retinol

Mineral Oil

Since efficient absorption of both β-carotene and retinol is dependent on the vitamin being in a micellar solution, it is not surprising that drugs which interfere with the formation of micelles may reduce absorption. Mineral oil, the first drug to be shown to interfere both with β-carotene and with retinol absorption, reduces β-carotene primarily because the carotene is dissolved in the mineral oil and subsequently excreted in the feces [8]. However, it has been suggested that another effect of mineral oil is to interfere with micelle formation and that this effect may explain the observed reduction in the absorption both of β-carotene and of retinol in people who consume large amounts of mineral oil.

Bile Acid Sequestrants

The bile acid sequestrants, cholestyramine and colestipol, have potential for inducing malabsorption of both β-carotene and vitamin A. These drugs not only promote the fecal excretion of bile acids, but also, in high dosage, cause steatorrhea [13]. A risk of β-carotene and retinol malabsorption has been defined. However, while indirect evidence of a drug-induced impairment of vitamin A absorption has been obtained, clinical evidence of vitamin A deficiency with long-term cholestyramine and colestipol therapy has either not been encountered or has not been reported. *Longenecker and Basu* [23] showed that in subjects given cholestyramine with vitamin A in olive oil, peak serum levels of retinol are less than when the same dose of oil is administered to control subjects not receiving the drug.

Prolonged treatment of familial hypercholesterolemia in children with cholestyramine causes a lowering of serum retinol and also of vitamin E levels [35]. A possibility exists, from our knowledge of nutrient factors influencing retinol absorption, that vitamin A and E malabsorption is interactive.

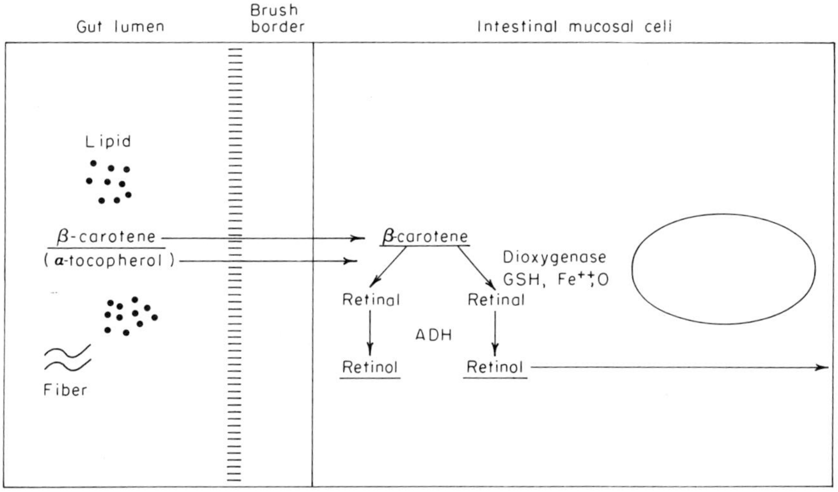

Fig. 1. β-Carotene absorption and conversion to retinol, showing location of interacting nutrients. GSH = Reduced glutathione; ADH = alcohol dehydrogenase.

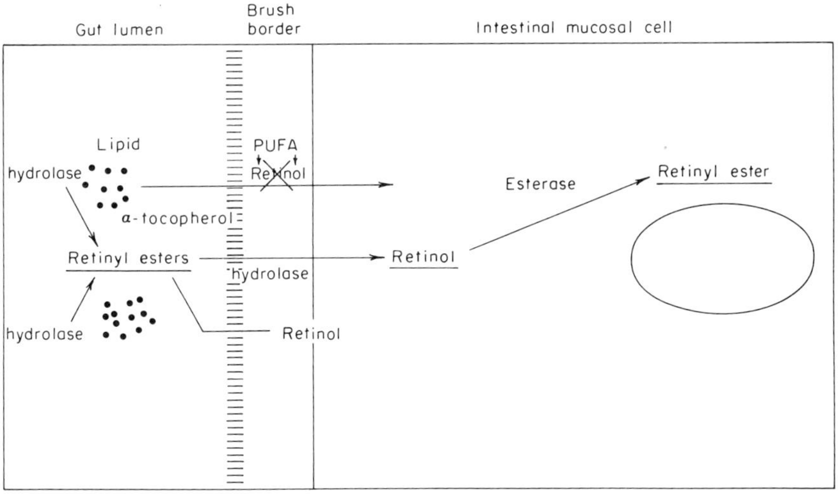

Fig. 2. Retinol absorption showing location of interacting nutrients. PUFA = Polyunsaturated fatty acids.

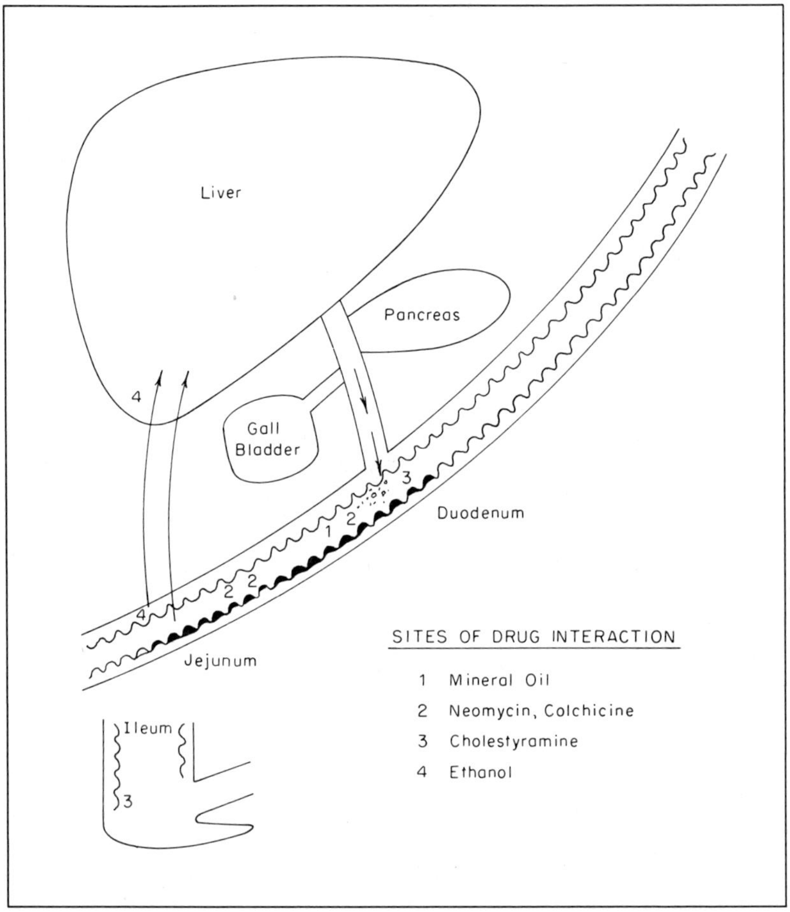

Fig. 3. Sites of action of drugs causing malabsorption of β-carotene and retinol.

Anti-Inflammatory Drugs

Reduced serum carotene levels and steatorrhea have been reported in patients receiving oral colchicine [27]. Colchicine causes acute intestinal mucosal injury with loss of integrity of the brush border. Interference with fat absorption and with absorption of fat-soluble vitamins is secondary to this mucosal damage.

Antibiotics

Neomycin has multiple effects which cause maldigestion and malabsorption. It causes intestinal mucosal injury but also precipitates fatty acids and, to a lesser extent, bile acids from bile salt-lipid micelles, so that the micellar phase in the small intestine is interrupted. This impairment of micelle formation and function may explain adverse effects of neomycin on the absorption of β-carotene and retinol [5, 10]. Drugs causing malabsorption of β-carotene and retinol and their sites as well as their mechanism of action are indicated in figure 3.

Riboflavin

Sources of the Vitamin

A brief resume of the sources of riboflavin which are ingested is a prerequisite for understanding factors which influence the bioavailability of the vitamin. Sources of riboflavin include conventional foods, enriched foods, formula foods, vitamin supplements, other nutrient supplements, and alcoholic beverages [14]. The form of riboflavin in these sources differs but may include free riboflavin (FR), riboflavin 5′-phosphate (flavin mononucleotide, FMN), flavin adenine dinucleotide (FAD), and flavin-containing peptides. A reference listing of riboflavin sources is given in table II which also shows which of these sources provide pharmacological as distinct from physiological or trace amounts of the vitamin. The form(s) of the vitamin in each source is designated. Milk contains free riboflavin. Most of the flavin present in food, other than milk, is in the form of the two flavin coenzymes.

Absorption

During the process of digestion the major part of these coenzymes is converted to free riboflavin. Rat studies show that in the digestive process there is a sequential hydrolysis of FMN and FAD by enzymes in the intestinal brush border and the flavin which is actually absorbed is free riboflavin. The brush border enzyme necessary to the hydrolysis of FMN and FAD are FMN phosphatase and FAD pyrophosphatase, respectively [2].

Riboflavin is absorbed by a specialized transport process from a specific saturable site in the proximal part of the small intestine [20]. While riboflavin is dephosphorylated at the brush border, after transport into the

Table II. Food, beverage, formula and pharmacological sources of riboflavin

Food (FMN, FAD, FR)	*Vitamin supplements*
M	M → H
A. Animal	A. riboflavin tablets
Milk – cheese	capsules (FR)
Eggs	B. multivitamin mixtures
Meat	(a) tablets (FR)
B. Plant	(b) liquid (FR)
Cereals: { enriched, unenriched	(c) injectable (FMN)
Fruit	*Other nutrient supplements*
Vegetables	M
	yeast
Formulas (FR, FMN)	*Alcoholic beverages*
M → H	L
A. Semisynthetic (polymeric)	A. wines (FR)
(a) Adult (FR)	B. beers (FR)
(b) Infant (FR)	
B. Synthetic (monomeric)	
(a) Enteral (FR)	
(b) Parenteral (FMN)	

H, M, L = Designating high, medium, low vitamin concentration.

mucosal cell, it is rephosphorylated. Enterohepatic circulation of riboflavin has been proposed and is supported by animal and human studies. After absorption, both riboflavin and FMN are transported in the plasma and a large fraction is bound to plasma proteins [18, 33].

Diet-Related Factors Which Influence Bioavailability

The bioavailability of pharmacological doses of riboflavin is influenced by the vitamer, the dose, and the form of the vitamin, as well as by the characteristic of the food, formula or beverage which may be consumed with the vitamin. It was shown by *Stewart* et al. [31] that the in vitro release of riboflavin from gelatin capsules is dependent on the vitamin diluent inside the capsule. Volunteers receiving capsules containing lactose absorbed more of the vitamin than those ingesting capsules containing kaolin as diluent.

In 1964, *Middleton* et al. [25] established a relationship between the in vitro disintegration and dissolution time of riboflavin tablets and showed a correlation with physiological availability of the vitamin. Physicochemical differences between free riboflavin and FMN, including greater solubility of the latter in aqueous media, influence the relative rates of absorption of equivalent doses of these vitamins [19].

The characteristics of the beverage which is drunk, when a solid formulation of riboflavin is taken, may affect the rate of absorption of the vitamin. We have recently demonstrated that when riboflavin tablets are given with a glucose polymer solution of the type used in enteral formulae, riboflavin absorption is slower than when the same dose of riboflavin is given with milk. This is explained by differential solubility of the riboflavin in the two beverages [6]. Bioavailability of riboflavin is increased by the glucose polymer.

Riboflavin availability is enhanced by dietary components and other diet characteristics which delay the rate of stomach emptying or affect intestinal transit. Larger meals, hot meals, and fat-containing meals all have this effect [16]. The net effect is to optimize the rate of delivery of riboflavin to its absorption site. Slow stomach emptying not only allows more time for disintegration of riboflavin in solid formulation, but also optimizes delivery of the riboflavin to the saturable absorption site.

Sodium alginate, which is used as a food additive to thicken dessert-type dairy products, promotes riboflavin availability, probably because it forms a viscous solution which moves through the gastrointestinal tract slowly so that the vitamin is retained longer at the absorption site [21]. Cola beverages which contain phosphoric acid and sugar increase riboflavin bioavailability because the soluble carbohydrate and the phosphoric acid both slow gastric emptying [7].

We have shown that certain dietary fiber sources also increase the bioavailability of riboflavin. The largest effect is obtained with coarse bran which reduces intestinal transit time but may slow the delivery of the vitamin from the stomach to the duodenum [28]. Dietary factors which influence riboflavin availability are shown in figure 4.

Drug Effects on the Availability of Riboflavin

Drugs which diminish the bioavailability of riboflavin may adsorb the vitamin within the gut lumen. Although clinical evidence is lacking to support this statement, it is presumed that medications containing kaolin could

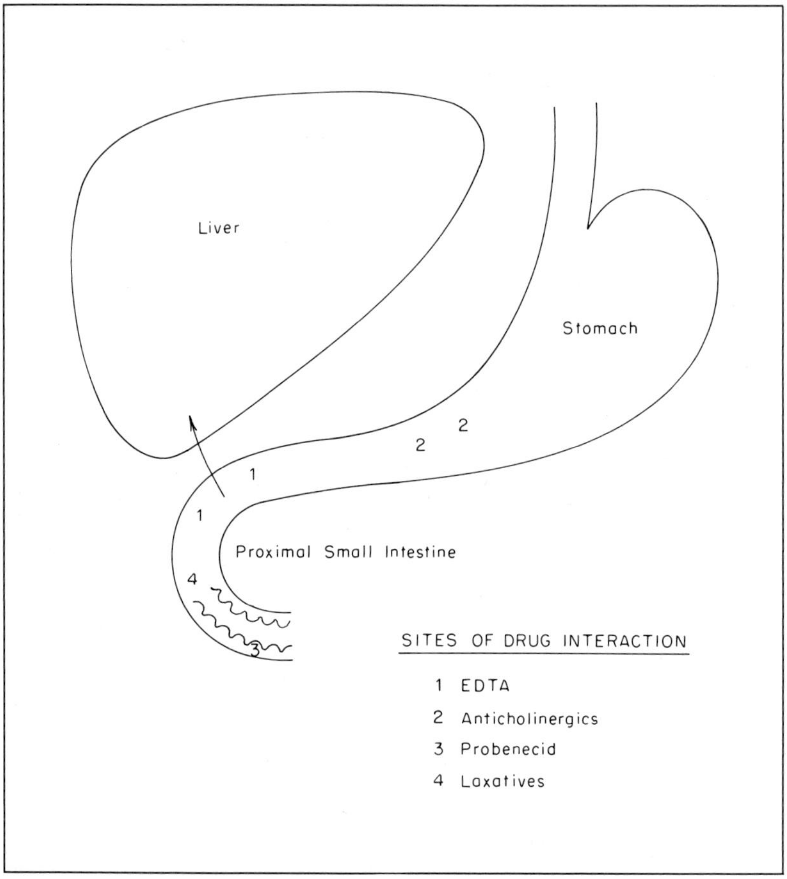

Fig. 4. Sites of action of drugs causing malabsorption of riboflavin.

decrease riboflavin absorption since kaolin, within riboflavin capsules, has this effect. Availability of flavin coenzymes may be reduced because of inhibition of the phosphatases at the brush border. Ethylenediaminetetra-acetic acid (EDTA) has been shown to inhibit FMN hydrolysis as well as FAD hydrolysis in vitro [2]. Whether EDTA, administered parenterally as a chelating agent in heavy metal poisoning, has this effect has not been documented but is likely. Few drugs have been clearly identified as having an inhibitory effect on riboflavin absorption. However, *Jusko and Levy* [17] provided indirect evidence that probenecid inhibits the specialized transport process responsible for the specialized transport intestinal absorption of riboflavin.

Drugs which increase the rate of stomach emptying or which cause intestinal hurry may diminish the time of occupancy of the vitamin at the site of absorption and therefore decrease the efficiency of riboflavin absorption. Thyroxine may have this effect, as proposed by *Levy* et al. [22].

Discussion

In this analysis of diet and drug effects on the bioavailability of pharmacological levels of model vitamins, main effects are seen to vary with the lipid or water solubility of the micronutrient. For fat-soluble vitamins, such as β-carotene, bioavailability is enhanced by diet and drug variables which promote passive transport, increase stability, and reduce gastrointestinal metabolism. However, absorption of the metabolite retinol, while being similarly related to food and drug factors which determine transport and stability, is also promoted by increased gastrointestinal metabolism of the parent compound.

On the other hand, bioavailability of water-soluble vitamins, such as riboflavin, is enhanced by diet and drug variables which promote dissolution of the vitamin preparation as well as those which reduce gastric emptying time and optimize delivery of the vitamin to the absorption site.

The likelihood that a food constituent or a drug will affect the bioavailability of these vitamins and the direction of the effect can therefore be predicted, knowing physicochemical and functional properties of the food or drug in question.

Parallels can also be drawn between effects of nutrients or non-nutrient food constituents on the availability of these model vitamins and the effects of the same food factors on the bioavailability of drugs which have a similar mode of absorption. Thus, the model vitamins are prototypes of lipid and water-soluble drugs with respect to major determinants of bioavailability. If a food constituent affects the bioavailability of one or another of these model vitamins it may have a similar effect on drugs which share absorption characteristics (table III). Exceptions to this generalization are related to specific properties of these vitamins which are not shared by drugs, such as specialized transport. However, evidence suggests that in man, food effects on the availability of these vitamins and on drugs which have similar biopharmaceutical or pharmacokinetic properties are alike.

Table III. Comparison between absorption characteristics of model vitamins and drugs and effects of food constituents on their bioavailability

Absorption characteristics	Vitamin	Drug	Constituent affecting food bioavailability
Micellar uptake	β-carotene	salicylamide [24]	fat ↑
Presystemic intestinal metabolism	retinol	propranolol [34]	protein ↑
Site-specific saturable process	riboflavin	chlorothiazide [26] hydrochlorothiazide	carbohydrate, fat ↑
Transport time-dependent	β-carotene	acetaminophen [15]	fiber ↑ (pectin)

References

1 Arnrich, L.; Arthur, V.A.: Interactions of fat soluble vitamins in hypervitaminoses. Ann. N.Y. Acad. Sci. *355:* 109–118 (1980).

2 Akiyama, T.; Selhub, J.; Rosenberg, I.H.: FMN phosphatase and FAD phosphatase in rat intestinal brush borders: role in intestinal absorption of dietary riboflavin. J. Nutr. *112:* 263–268 (1982).

3 Barnard, D.L.; Heaton, K.W.: Bile acids and vitamin A absorption in man. The effect of two bile acid binding agents, cholestyramine and lignin. Gut *14:* 316–318 (1973).

4 Barrowman, J.A.: Drug effects on fat soluble vitamin absorption; in Hathcock, Coon, Nutrition and drug interrelations, pp. 113–130 (Academic Press, New York 1978).

5 Barrowman, J.; D'Mello, A.; Herxheimer, A.: A single dose of neomycin impairs absorption of vitamin A (retinol) in man. Eur. J. clin. Pharmacol. *5:* 199–202 (1973).

6 Belko, A.Z.: Personal communication (1982).

7 Brian Houston, J.; Levy, G.: Effect of carbonated beverages and of an antiemetic containing carbohydrate and phosphoric acid on riboflavin bioavailability and salicylamide biotransformation in humans. J. pharm. Sci. *64:* 1504–1507 (1975).

8 Curtis, A.C.; Ballmer, R.S.: The prevention of carotene absorption by liquid petrolatum. J. Am. med. Ass. *113:* 1785–1788 (1939).

9 El-Gorab, M.J.; Underwood, B.A.; Loerch, J.: The roles of bile salts in the uptake of beta-carotene and retinol by rat everted gut sacs. Biochim. biophys. Acta *401:* 265–277 (1975).

10 Faloon, W.W.: Drug production of intestial malabsorption. N.Y. State J. Med. *70:* 2189–2191 (1970).

11 Goodman, W.S. De; Huang, H.S.: Biosynthesis of vitamin A with rat intestinal enzyme. Science *149:* 879–880 (1965).
12 Gronowska-Senger, A.; Smaczny, E.; Dobkowicz, B.: The effect of fiber on the utilization of carotene in laboratory rats. Bromatol. Chemia Toksykologiczna *13:* 129–134 (1980).
13 Hashim, S.A.; Bergen, S.S.; Van Itallie, T.B.: Experimental steatorrhea induced in man by bile acid sequestrant. Proc. Soc. exp. Biol. Med. *106:* 173–175 (1961).
14 Hunt, S.M.: Nutritional intake of riboflavin; in Rivlin, Riboflavin, pp. 199–219 (Plenum Press, New York 1975).
15 Jaffe, J.M.; Coliazzi, J.L.; Barry, H.: Effects of dietary components on gastrointestinal absorption of acetaminophen tablets in man. J. pharm. Sci. *60:* 1646–1650 (1971).
16 Jusko, W.J.; Levy, G.: Absorption, metabolism and excretion of riboflavin 5′-phosphate in man. J. pharm. Sci. *56:* 58–62 (1967).
17 Jusko, W.J.; Levy, G.: Effect of probenecid on riboflavin absorption and excretion in man. J. pharm. Sci. *56:* 1145–1149 (1967).
18 Jusko, W.J.; Levy, G.: Plasma protein binding of riboflavin and riboflavin 5′-phosphate in man. J. pharm. Sci. *58:* 58–62 (1969).
19 Jusko, W.J.; Levy, G.: Absorption, protein binding and elimination of riboflavin; in Rivlin, Riboflavin, pp. 99–151 (Plenum Press, New York 1975).
20 Levy, G.; Jusko, W.J.: Factors affecting the absorption of riboflavin in man. J. pharm. Sci. *55:* 285–289 (1966).
21 Levy, G.; Rao, B.K.: Enhanced intestinal absorption of riboflavin from sodium alginate solution in man. J. pharm. Sci. *61:* 279–280 (1972).
22 Levy, G.; MacGillray, M.N.; Procknal, J.A.: Riboflavin absorption in children with thyroid disorders. Pediatrics, Springfield *50:* 896–900 (1972).
23 Longenecker, J.B.; Basu, S.G.: Effect of cholestyramine on absorption of amino acids and vitamin A in man (Abstract). Fed. Proc. *24:* 375 (1965).
24 Morad, A.R.M.: Salicylamide pharmacokinetics in healthy males: dietary effect. Biopharmaceut. Drug Dispos. *3:* 175–183 (1982).
25 Middleton, E.J.; Davies, J.M.; Morrison, A.B.: Relationship between rate of dissolution disintegration time and physiological availability of riboflavin in sugar coated tablets. J. pharm. Sci. *53:* 1378–1380 (1964).
26 Osman, M.A.; Patel, R.B.; Irwin, D.S.; Graig, W.A.; Welling, P.G.: Bioavailability of chlorothiazide from 50, 100, and 250 mg solution doses. Biopharmaceut. Drug Dispos. *3:* 89–94 (1982).
27 Race, T.F.; Paes, I.C.; Faloon, W.W.: Intestinal malabsorption induced by oral colchicine. Comparison with neomycin and cathartic agents. Am. J. med. Sci. *259:* 32–41 (1970).
28 Roe, D.A.; Wrick, K.; McLain, D.; Van Soest, P.: Effects of dietary fiber sources on riboflavin absorption. Fed. Proc. *37:* 756 (1978).
29 Roels, O.A.; Trout, M.; Dujacquier, R.: Carotene balances of boys in Ruanda where vitamin A deficiency is prevalent. J. Nutr. *65:* 115–127 (1958).
30 Sivakumar, B.; Reddy, V.: Absorption of labeled vitamin A in children during infection. Br. J. Nutr. *27:* 229–304 (1972).
31 Stewart, A.G.; Grant, D.J.W.; Newton, J.M.: The release of a model low dose drug (riboflavine) from hard gelatin capsule for mutations. J. Pharm. Pharmac. *31:* 1–6 (1976).

32 Stoecker, B.; Arnrich, L.: Patterns of protein feeding and the biosynthesis of vitamin A from carotene in rats. J. Nutr. *103:* 1112–1118 (1973).
33 Stripp, B.: Intestinal absorption of riboflavin in man. Acta pharmac. tox. *22:* 353–362 (1965).
34 Walle, T.; Fagan, T.C.; Walle, U.K.; Oexman, M.-J.; Conradi, E.C.; Gaffney, T.E.: Food-induced increase in propranolol bioavailability. Relationship to protein and effects on metabolites. Clin. Pharmacol. Ther. *30:* 790–795 (1981).
35 West, R.J.; Lloyd, J.K.: The effect of cholestyramine on intestinal absorption. Gut *16:* 93–98 (1975).
36 Wolf, G.: Vitamin A; in Alfin-Slater, Kritchevsky, Human nutrition: a comprehensive treatise, vol. 3B, pp. 97–203 (Plenum Press, New York 1980).
37 Zachman, R.D.; Olson, J.A.: Uptake of ^{14}C-β-carotene and its conversion to retinol ester by the isolated perfused rat liver. J. biol. Chem. *238:* 541–546 (1963).

Prof. D.A. Roe, Division of Nutritional Sciences, Cornell University, Ithaca, NY 14853 (USA)

Wld Rev. Nutr. Diet., vol. 43, pp. 95–116 (Karger, Basel 1984)

Nutrition and Drug-Protein Binding

André Gayte-Sorbier, Charles B. Airaudo

Laboratoire de Bromatologie, Diététique et Analyse appliquée à l'Expertise, Faculté de Pharmacie, Marseille, France

Plasma protein binding of drugs plays a major role in the modulation of their pharmacological action. The present work reviews how nutrition can affect the activity of drugs via such a phenomenon. At this stage, that is after the absorption of the drug molecules and their release in the circulation, a direct interaction is unthinkable between nutrients and drugs. Possible interferences may occur only via protein-drug-bindings on the one hand and protein-nutrient or more generally protein-biological molecule bindings on the other hand. Among these molecules, 'free' fatty acids (FFA) are likely to play an outstanding role through their action on protein-drug bindings. The nutritional state itself, however, may also intervene because of its influence on the circulating level of FFA although the ingestion of lipids is not essential to it. Figure 1 illustrating schematically possible interactions endeavors to show the role as intermediates of protein bindings.

Binding Properties of Proteins [5]

Almost only binding to serum albumin will be dealt with in the present work. It would, however, be wrongly assumed to be the only one capable of binding: drugs can also be bound more particularly by α- and β-lipoproteins but to a lesser extent. This is observed, although not exclusively, at toxic dose levels: the drug 'colonizes' gradually the various proteins as it is released in the circulation. It would also be wrong to believe that albumin binds only to drugs or nutrients. Its binding capacity also concerns cations, anions such as fatty acids and many biological substances (tryptophan, bilirubin, bile acids, steroid hormones, thyroxin, etc.).

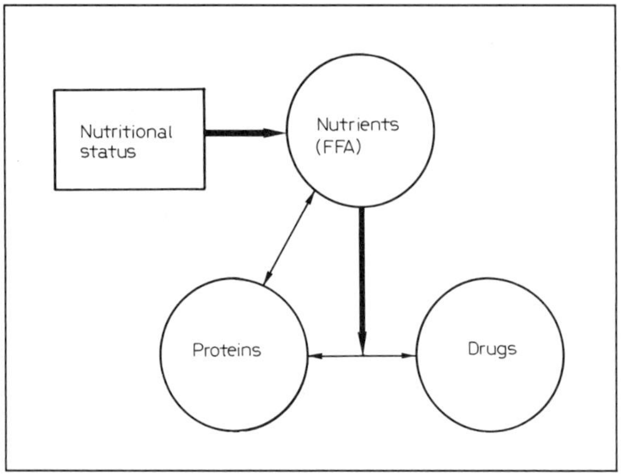

Fig. 1. Schematic illustration of food and drug interactions.

The structures of human and bovine albumins are closely related. This permitted to conduct many studies on bovine albumin on account of its lower cost. They differ in the number of amino acids (584 or 585 according to the authors and 581 for human and bovine albumins, respectively) and in the nature of some of them and subsequently in their molecular weight (66,248 and 66,210, respectively). The binding capacity being essentially associated with the tertiary structure, these differences in primary structure are probably unimportant in the present case. The results of the in vitro studies are likely to be extrapolable from one albumin to another. On the contrary, such extrapolation is not necessarily licit in other animal species. It seems in particular difficult and even impossible to predict binding in man from in vivo experiments in the species routinely used.

The molecule of albumin is composed of a single long chain, folded in 9 double loops resulting from disulfide bridges built on Cys-Cys groups. The large (L) and small (S) loops are distributed according to the repeated sequence LSL-LSL-LSL corresponding to loops 1,2,3–4,5,6–7,8,9, respectively.

In hydrodynamic studies, the molecule was shown at plasma pH value to present a prolate compact ellipsoidal shape, probably due to important attraction forces between certain loops. The tertiary structure develops inside this 'shell'. Since 1966, this structure has been proposed to result from an association of loops in three globular, spherical parts, joined together linearly and called 'domains' (fig. 2). Studies on the polarization of the fluorescence of the complexes formed with 1-anilino-8-naphthylsulfonic acid suggest the existence of four binding sites with a strong affinity for the organic molecules in the hydrophobic intervals at the junctions of the central sphere and of the two outer ones. Each junction therefore corresponds to two binding sites.

According to more recent studies (1975), the tertiary structure would be composed of 3 cylindrical domains. Each one consists of 5 parallel helices. The major binding sites would then be located in holes or pockets inside and not between the 3 domains as in the model above. The first domain corresponds approximately to loops 1,2,3 (exactly to residues 1–191), the second one to loops 4,5,6 (residues 192–384) and the third one to loops 7,8,9 (residues 385–584).

These conclusions are based on recent works involving partial hydrolyses with various enzymes at different pH values. For instance, pepsin cleaves bovine albumin between residues 306 and 307 into two fragments, each of them corresponding to one of the outer domains and to one part of the central one. Each fragment presents qualitatively the same binding potential towards C_8- and C_{16}-saturated fatty acids, towards bilirubin and various organic dyes. This suggests that the outer domains bear the binding sites of the large organic molecules. The sum of the binding capacities of the fragments remains, however, below that of intact albumin. Combining both fractions is sufficient to restore the initial binding capacity except towards the C_{16} fatty acid. It seems that the cleavage would destroy other sites which ensure the binding of a number of organic compounds. Consequently sites would also be present in the central domain.

Independently of any experimental consideration, the notion of binding site is furthermore justified from a theoretical or even intuitive viewpoint. The molecular weight (MW) of drugs does not generally exceed 300. These molecules are small compared to albumin (MW, 66,000). Drugs bind exclusively to very small surfaces of the albumin molecule which are the binding sites. When several sites exist for the same compound, their affinities differ. Number *n* of binding sites corresponds to the maximum number of moles bound per mole of albumin.

Thanks especially to studies on binding carried out on isolated fragments, attempts were made to assign a position to the binding sites of several compounds (fig. 2). Some positions seem to be determined, in particular the binding sites of nickel and copper on the thiol group of the Cys_{34} residue towards the amine end of the chain. An important binding site of

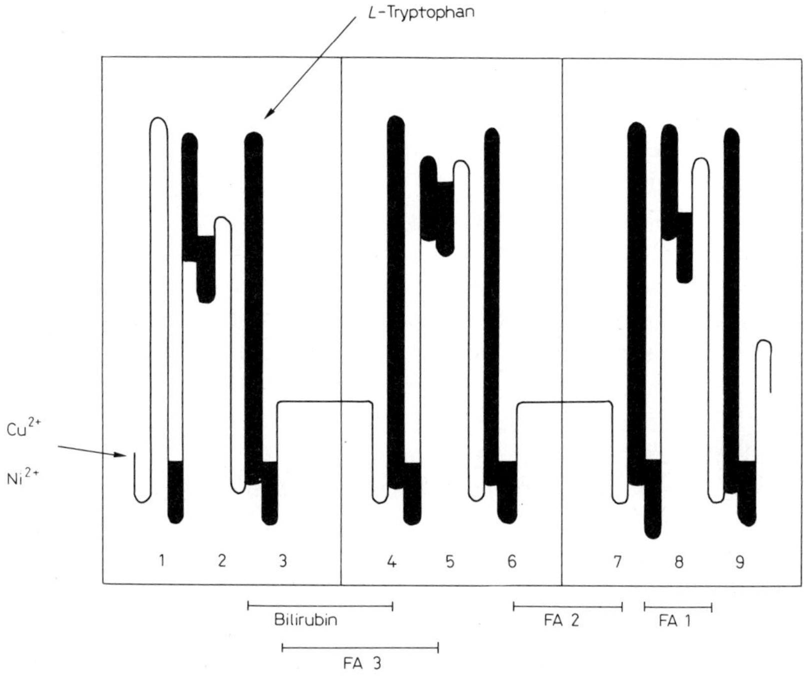

Fig. 2. The three domains of the albumin molecule and their binding sites [according to ref. 5] (FA = fatty acids).

fatty acids with long and medium chains is located at the carboxyl end towards loops 7–8, between residues 377 and 503. It is therefore probably associated with the third domain. A second less definite site of fatty acids is present between loops 6 and 7. A third weaker site would be located towards loop 4, thus permitting interference of fatty acids with the binding of tryptophan and bilirubin in the cleft between loops 3 and 4. Aspirin is believed to bind in the same region.

Characteristics of the Drug-Albumin Binding [15]

The only drugs which do not bind to plasma proteins are small water-soluble molecules such as glucose, ouabain, nicotinic acid, isoniazid, etc. The other drugs form reversible protein combinations which ensure their transfer in the circulation. These combinations which are not able to cross the cell membranes are pharmacologically inactive. This binding process of drugs to proteins results in a modulation of their activity. Indeed if the drug-protein combination is very steady, the drug will remain partially or transiently in the circulation in the inactive state. It will be released only in those tissues likely to substitute for the initial plasma combination steadier tissue combinations, or at least as steady ones. Inversely, if the plasma binding is endowed with only a very low stability the drug will be massively and rapidly distributed in the tissues. Plasma proteins are therefore drug acceptors which, via the transient storage they ensure, induce a physiological sustained-release effect. Pharmacokinetically speaking, it results in a small distribution volume and in a large half-life time.

The mass law is the major factor in this equilibrium:

$$[\text{Free, active drug}] + [\text{Free protein}] \underset{k_2}{\overset{k_1}{\rightleftarrows}} [\text{Bound, inactive drug}].$$

k_1 and k_2 are respectively the formation and dissociation rate constants of the combination. Their ratio:

$$Ka = \frac{k_1}{k_2}$$

is the association constant. It corresponds to the affinity of the drug for the protein considered and, at equilibrium, is equal to:

$$\frac{[\text{Bound drug}]}{[\text{Free drug}] \times [\text{Free protein}]} = \frac{k_1}{k_2}.$$

In the equation above, the concentrations are expressed in molarity, *M*. The association constant and the affinity are thus expressed in M^{-1} (as $M/M^2 = M^{-1}$) or in liter/mol. The association constants reported in the literature for different drugs range from 5×10^2 to 4×10^5 M^{-1}.

The drug-protein combinations generally proceed from hydrogen, ionic or electrostatic bonds or from Van der Waals' forces, very rarely from covalence (such is, however, the case of aspirin capable of forming acetylalbumin). The hydrogen bonds are frequently strengthened by a 'hydrophobic' bond, that is resulting from an interaction between nonpolar groups [11].

Classically, drug fall into two categories according to their form of bond. The weak acid molecules of pK_a ranging from 3.5 to 6.0 and in consequence completely or almost completely ionized at plasma pH value have in common a group of sites with strong affinity. The number of these sites varies between 0.6 and 2.5. The difference between these values is not very surprising (at first sight such a difference may seem contrary to common sense as these sites are common to the whole group of drugs), neither is their fractional nature. First the binding is only a probability but not a certainty. Moreover, the molecule of albumin does not present constantly the same spatial configuration because of its flexibility. Finally, the spatial configurations of both partners at the very time of the binding also intervene. However, it should be kept in mind that obtaining a fractional number of sites during the experimentation may originate in the presence of a form of albumin having lost some binding sites. This induces an error in the binding protein concentration.

Some weak acid drug molecules have moreover a second group of binding sites with a lower affinity. The number of these sites varies between 3 and 4.

These ionized molecules bind via ionic bonds strengthened by a hydrophobic bond in the case of the first group of sites. They have only a limited number of sites. Their binding depends on the albumin concentration and on the presence of competitors, that is molecules of therapeutic or biological origin with the same binding site. The binding of this type of drug is illustrated by the case of warfarin (pK_a 5.1): the number of sites is limited since the percentage of binding decreases while the warfarin concentration increases (fig. 3a). However, the affinity is strong since the percentage of binding at low drug concentrations is high when albumin is in excess (fig. 3b).

The case of drugs with pK_a between 7 and 9, thus poorly ionized in plasma, is almost the reverse. They are weak bases or very weak acids (barbiturates). Nonionizable molecules also belong to this category (digitoxin). Imipramine (pK_a 9.5) illustrates this: the percentage of binding remains steady whereas its concentration increases (fig. 3a). This shows that the amount bound increases proportionally and consequently that the number of sites is large, but the affinity is low, since the initial percentage of binding is relatively low in the presence of an albumin excess (fig. 3b). This second category of drugs is hydrogen-bound forming 'hydrophobic' bonds. In the present case only a single group of sites exists. The number of sites per molecule of albumin may exceed 30. Accordingly, competitions for the occupation of the sites are unlikely in such a case.

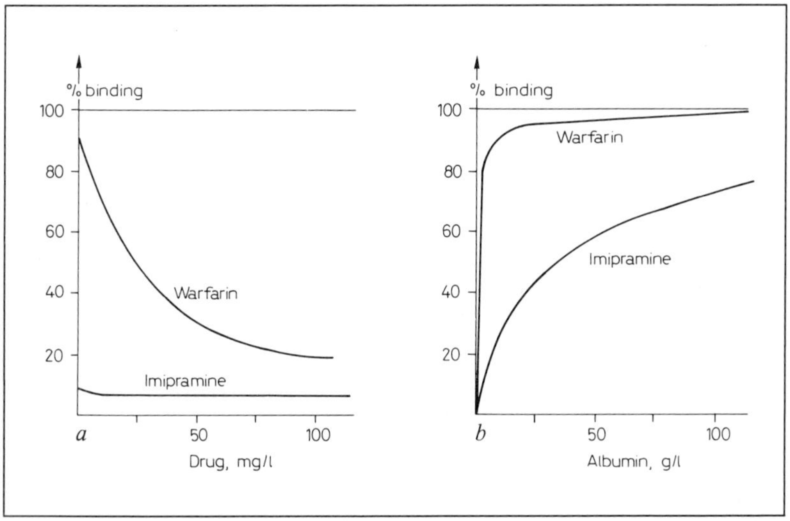

Fig. 3. Determination of the albumin binding characteristics of a drug [according to ref. 15]. *a* Constant albumin concentration (2 g/l). *b* Constant drug concentrations (0.1 μg/ml).

Effects of Nutrition on Drug-Protein Binding

The phenomenon of drug plasma binding described above may be affected by nutrition via two mechanisms: one involves plasma protein concentrations, the other plasma fatty acid concentrations.

Influence of Protein Concentrations

In protein-calorie malnutrition states such as kwashiorkor, a drastic decrease in plasma albumin levels is observed: a deficiency in sites available for the binding of drugs exists. At a given concentration of drug, the amount bound is inferior to what it would be in normal subjects. The concentration in active form being higher, the drug is found to diffuse massively in the tissues. Its pharmacological effect is intensified but its elimination accelerated. However, this hypothesis is rare in wealthy countries in which the individual binding variations due to proteins are minor and appear to result essentially, apart from pathological circumstances inducing hypoalbuminemia, from the very structure of albumin, i.e. from genetic factors. Moreover, this question does not seem to have been much investigated in underdeveloped countries. However, a few studies have been carried out recently in India.

These studies showed that in undernourished subjects with concomitant hypoalbuminemia, plasma binding of tetracycline was significantly reduced [12]. Later on a pharmacokinetic study confirmed this conclusion by comparing the metabolism of drug in normal (albuminemia: 4.2 g/dl) and undernourished (albuminemia: 3.2 g/dl) subjects [8]. Plasma concentrations with time were found to decrease more rapidly in undernourished subjects. The distribution of tetracycline was improved because of the reduced percentage of binding resulting from the protein deficiency. However, other phenomena irrelevant to the present subject were also involved.

On the contrary, another comparative study on streptomycin in normal (albuminemia: 4.2 g/dl) and undernourished (albuminemia: 2.9 g/dl) subjects showed that the plasma concentration reached was identical but occurred only after 1 h in undernourished subjects instead of 30 min in normal subjects [7]. The percentages of binding were comparable in the two groups (57.3 and 61.9% in vitro, 48.4 and 47.3% in vivo) in spite of hypoalbuminemia. Tetracycline was thought to bind almost exclusively to albumin whereas according to the results of a previous study [1] the binding of streptomycin would involve albumin only for approximately 50% of the whole bound fraction. The remaining streptomycin would be bound to globulins. Total proteinemias being identical in the two groups of subjects, this would explain the similarity of the binding percentages in the two groups in spite of the concomitant hypoalbuminemia in the undernourished group. However, according to other studies, the binding of tetracycline would involve albumin only for a little more than 50% of the whole bound fraction [17].

Influence of Free Fatty Acid Concentrations

The second mechanism by which nutrition may interfere with the plasma protein binding of drugs consists in its effects on the circulating level of metabolites or endogenous biological molecules likely to occupy competitively the binding sites of drugs.

The albumin binding of such substances has already been briefly reviewed: bilirubin, bile acids, nonpolar amino acids such as tryptophan, FFA, steroids, thyroxin, etc. Actually, hormones and substances with vitamin action (of biological or therapeutic origin) as well as synthetic molecules of chemically related structures are carried in the circulation by specific proteins such as corticosteroid binding globulin (CBG) in the case of glucocorticoids or cortisol, testosterone estradiol binding globulin (TEBG) in the case of androgens or estrogens, or thyroxin binding globulin (TBG) in the case of thyroxin. This specific binding is characterized by a limited number of binding sites but a strong affinity. Then albumin makes only an accessory binding (when the specific proteins become saturated) characterized on the contrary by a larger number of sites but less affinity. Competition between such acid biological substances and weak acid drugs, for the occupation on albumin of the binding sites of the latter, is not necessarily to be ruled out. These sites are not specific of drugs. Such are the differences of affinity, however, that the drugs generally override the others. (The hypocholesterolemic activity of clofibrate would result, at least partly, from the fact that its major metabolite, chlorophenoxyisobutyric acid, binds to albumin, thus displacing the initially bound thyroxin, releasing it and allowing its diffusion in the tissues, in particular at the liver level in which it increases the catabolism of cholesterol.)

Although the circulating levels of such biological molecules may be affected by nutrition, it is not realistic to refer to an interference of nutrition with the binding of drugs and subsequently with their activity. These competitions might, nevertheless, have therapeutic consequences under certain physiological or pathological circumstances. The binding of ionized drugs decreases during pregnancy, probably because of the hormone binding, or in subjects under stress with higher fatty acid levels.

Actually it seems that the only biological substances likely to affect drug binding are FFA. FFA are also nutrients but fatless food intake may also influence drug-protein binding via FFA because of the intricacy of the various metabolisms involved.

Free Fatty Acids and Their Binding to Albumin. The object of the present work is not to describe in detail the metabolism of FFA which would bring us to develop a large part of the metabolism of lipids in general. It will only be specified that: the time-honored term ‘free’ actually means ‘nonesterified’, fatty acids being inevitably bound to plasma albumin which ensures their transfer in the circulation; these FFA have a double origin, each of them being related to the nutritional state.

FFA first result from the hydrolysis of triglycerides of plasma lipoproteins (essentially chylomicrons of intestinal origin and very low density lipoproteins (VLDL) of intestinal and hepatic origin, both following the ingestion of lipids). During the postprandial period, FFA constitute a form of very transient but compulsory transfer between food lipids and tissues, either adipose tissue in which they are stored or muscles of the skeleton and heart at the level of which they are directly used as a source of energy. The second origin of plasma FFA is precisely the lipolysis of triglycerides in the adipose tissue in case of energetic needs. During the postprandial period characterized by important levels of glucose and insulin, fatty acids were stored in the adipose tissue as triglycerides. They are on the contrary released in the form of FFA during periods of fast characterized by low circulating levels of glucose and insulin. This lipolysis is enhanced by glucagon, adrenaline or noradrenaline. Beside the nutritional viewpoint, the last point explains the increase in FFA levels in subjects under stress because of the stimulation of the sympathetic nerve ends.

The FFA fraction of plasma contains approximately 90% of 16- or 18-carbon atom acids. These long-chained FFA are believed to be ionized at plasma pH. They are 'fatty anions' which bind to albumin essentially via nonpolar bonds or incidentally via electrostatic bonds. The major form of bond is an insertion of the long fatty chains into the nonpolar pockets of the tertiary structure of albumin either in the holes between the spherical surfaces or inside the cylindrical domains according to the albumin structure accepted. As to human albumin, the association constants of palmitate ($C_{16:0}$) and oleate ($C_{18:1}$) were 6.2×10^7 and 2.6×10^8 M^{-1} respectively for the binding of the first mole and in the absence of dimerization or other forms of fatty chain association. Such constants are 150,000–520,000 times larger than those reported previously for drugs (5×10^2 to 4×10^5 M^{-1}). Although they are lower, the association constants corresponding to the following steps are however superior to those of drugs (table I). These anions of fatty acids therefore compete with drugs for albumin binding.

It is obvious that FFA can interfere with the plasma binding of drugs behaving similarly, that is drugs ionized at blood pH. However, although the binding of poorly ionized drugs is not altered at therapeutic dose levels by the presence of ionized molecules, the albumin binding of large amounts of fatty acids reduces that of a number of weak bases [15]. This phenomenon is still unclear to date.

As it is a competition between FFA and drugs for the occupation of the albumin sites, the problem can be put in terms of strength ratio, that is not only in terms of affinity but also of concentration. Nevertheless, before determining the level from which FFA are likely to interfere, it should be specified under which circumstances and within which limits the normal level may vary.

Table I. Association constants of the two more abundant FFA in plasma [according to ref. 14]

Ka	Palmitate (C_{16}), M^{-1}	Oleate (C_{18}), M^{-1}
Ka_1	6.2×10^7	2.6×10^8
Ka_2	2.3×10^7	9.4×10^7
Ka_3	1.2×10^7	2.9×10^7
Ka_4	3.1×10^6	2.1×10^7

Considering the rapidity of the mechanisms involved in the metabolism of fatty acids, plasma FFA concentrations may vary a lot over a short time. After an overnight fast, glucose administered orally (1 g/kg of body weight) decreases FFA levels by 60–75% within 1 h. This decrease already reaches 50% within 30 min. The disappearance rate of FFA is about 1.2 µEq/l/min. On the contrary, a fatty meal can more than double the FFA levels within 12 h. A fast observed for 39 h triples this level.

On the basis of the normal limits of these two biological parameters, the FFA/albumin molar ratio averaged 0.94 in venous blood of normal subjects at rest, with variations ranging from 0.46 to 1.75. This ratio is normally below 2. It exceeds this value only under special circumstances: e.g. prolonged physical exercise, i.v. administration of heparin to hypertriglyceridemic subjects (heparin is the co-factor of lipoprotein lipase, the enzyme responsible for the hydrolysis of plasma chylomicrons and VLDL) may increase the molar ratio up to 4.2. The only relevant situations in the present case are the postprandial period or fast. In fasting subjects, the values of the molar ratio range from 1.67 to 2.83. Under any circumstance, when the ratio exceeds 2, FFA begin to bind to supports other than albumin such as lipoproteins or erythrocytes.

The possibility of competition may be considered not only in quantitative terms. The fact that part of FFA results directly from the hydrolysis of plasma lipoproteins which are induced by the digestion of lipids establishes a direct relationship between the composition of the fats ingested and that of plasma FFA. The linoleic fraction of plasma FFA rises from 15 to 45% within 6 h after ingestion of safflower oil. This suggests that a single fatty meal is sufficient to change the composition of FFA, which may bring about consequences on the drug-protein bindings. If FFA can really interfere with these bindings such interference may depend not only on the FFA concentrations but also on their qualitative composition, thus on the type of fats consumed. A recent study which will be reviewed thereafter confirmed this hypothesis [6].

Studies Previously Conducted. Studies on the interference of FFA in the plasma protein binding of drugs can be divided into two periods. The first period which dates back over 30 years is characterized by in vitro studies mostly on organic dyes or fluorescent organic molecules simulating drugs, this for obvious assay facilities. This period is also characterized by a long stagnation following the preliminary evidence for this phenomenon. The second period still prevailing corresponds to the publication of various studies also carried out in vitro but with real drug molecules on the occasion of pharmacokinetic trials, as well as to entirely in vivo studies to determine the influence of food intake on drug binding. There is of course nothing absolute about these chronological considerations.

What follows is devoted to the analysis of several recent works. However, it is useful to dwell on previous studies as they are the basis of interpretations concerning the mechanism of action of fatty acids.

In vitro Studies

The first experimental study dealt with the binding of an organic dye, methylorange [14]. Like those of many drugs, the molecule of methylorange is large-sized because of the two aromatic cycles characterizing its structure. Its association constant with albumin is about 100 times lower than those of the first 2 mol of fatty acids bound. It is therefore comparable with those of drugs. It was shown that FFA displaced methylorange from its combination with human or bovine albumin but only when 2 mol of FFA were present.

Another work showed by the equilibrium dialysis method that not less than 3 mol of fatty acids were necessary to displace 1-anilino-8-naphthyl sulfonate (ANS) from human or bovine albumin: the displacement ranges from 15 to 20% [14]. Nevertheless, in the case of the bovine albumin-ANS complex, a significant fluorescence reduction was observed at FFA/albumin molar ratios below 3. Whereas at a ratio of 3, fluorescence was reduced by 15–28% thus in agreement with the results of equilibrium dialysis, the reduction already reached 3–10% at a molar ratio of 1 and 7–21% at a molar ratio of 2. These results were obtained with 12- to 18-carbon atom acids. The spectrum was qualitatively unchanged. In the case of the human albumin-ANS complex, fluorescence variations were also noted at molar ratios of 1 and 2. But, in contrast with what was observed with bovine albumin, fluorescence was more intense at these ratios than when albumin was poorer in fatty acids. The spectrum was qualitatively unchanged once more.

Another organic molecule used to simulate drug binding was 2-(4′-hydroxyphenylazo)benzoic acid (HABA) [14]. Bovine albumin binding of this compound caused a shift of its absorption peak from 380 to 480 nm. The optical density at the latter wavelength was therefore correlated with the amount bound. No influence could be shown by the equilibrium dialysis method at a molar ratio below 3, but optical density was reduced by 16% at 480 nm with palmitate at a ratio of 2. The absorbance reduction reached 38% at a ratio of 3. This might be considered to be in agreement with the percentage of decrease in binding determined by dialysis (15–25%). In the case of HABA and human albumin, a progressive shift of absorption peak towards the longer wavelengths was noted as the palmitate/albumin molar ratio increased.

In parallel with these experiments using dyes or fluophores, studies by the equilibrium dialysis method were conducted on radiolabeled drug molecules: salicylate, phenylbutazone, sulfadiazine, thiopental, and bishydroxycoumarin [14]. Addition of 3.5 or 7 mol of palmitate clearly reduced drug binding. However, no significant difference was observed below 3.5 mol of fatty acids. The same method applied to halofenate showed a reduction of binding by 15–30% when the molar ratio reached 3 [14]. Because of the scattered results, it was not possible to assess clearly a potential influence of palmitate at lower ratios. The reduction of binding in the latter cases might range from 5 to 10% at most.

In a work comparing plasma binding of valproic acid in normal subjects and subjects with liver diseases, the competition exerted by palmitate was studied in vitro by equilibrium dialysis with a radiolabeled molecule [16]. The palmitate/albumin molar ratios were approximately equal to 1, 2 and 3. The binding of valproic acid was inhibited proportionally to palmitate concentrations. At a drug concentration equal to 100 mg/l, the free fraction rose from 10 to 15%, then to 18% and finally to 22% when the molar ratio rose from 0 to 0.5, then to 1 and finally to 1.5. Although this study did not take into account the incidence of the nutritional state, it seems reasonable to conclude that the variations in FFA circulating levels in relation to the nutritional state would have the same effects.

The study on the in vitro binding of haloperidol was likewise based on the determination of its plasma levels in schizophrenic patients [9]. In a lipid-free serum, the free fraction of haloperidol was close to 10%. It remained almost steady when sodium oleate was added to lipid-free serum as long as the oleate/albumin molar ratio did not exceed 4. Beyond this value, the binding decreased, the free fraction reaching 17% when the ratio was equal to 8. In spite of the conclusion reported in the present work, variations in fatty acid levels such as those resulting from the nutritional state would thus not seem to have an incidence on the binding of haloperidol.

An in vitro study on the binding of three cephalosporin antibiotics can also be reported [6]. Its nature is strictly theoretical and general as it studied the influence of fatty acids with very different chain lengths and several of their derivatives which are normally not present in serum. But it led to relevant conclusions on the type of binding of FFA. It concerns all serum proteins as it was carried out on serum. The three drugs were selected for their differences in the extent of their binding although they were structurally related: moderately bound cephalothin, highly bound cefazolin, and even more bound cefonicid. When an inhibition of the binding was observed, it was at a fatty acids/proteins molar ratio which equalled or exceeded 3. Such an inhibition was all the more important as this ratio was higher. Among saturated acids, the most potent inhibitors were those containing 10–14 carbon atoms. The longest or shortest chains clearly hindered binding to a lesser extent. Maximum inhibition was obtained with a C_{10} chain for cephalothin, C_{10} or C_{12} chain for cefazolin (fig. 4) and C_{12} chain for cefonicid. In other words, palmitic acid which is normally one of the most abundant fatty acids in serum has a lower inhibitory potency compared with the shorter chain acids. On the other hand, the inhibition is all the more marked as the normal binding percentage of drugs is higher in the absence of inhibitors. The introduction of double bonds in the chains containing 16–18 carbon atoms increases the inhibitory potency. For instance, the difference in the bindings observed with and without fatty acids in the case of cefazolin rose from 34% with palmitic acid ($C_{16:0}$) to 50% with palmitoleic acid ($C_{16:1}$), and from 9% with stearic acid ($C_{18:0}$) to 42, 54 and 47%, respectively, with oleic ($C_{18:1}$), linoleic ($C_{18:2}$) and linolenic acid ($C_{18:3}$). Among the substituted derivatives studied, the sodium salts of lauric and oleic acids, i.e. fatty acid anions, had an inhibitory effect which was almost as intense as that of acids, which is logical. However, alcohols, chlorides, methyl esters, triglycerides and thiols did not inhibit the binding.

The last two results concerning the unsaturated chains and the substituted derivatives suggest that the inhibition varies according to the lipophilicity degree of the inhibitor: indeed unsaturation enhances inhibition whereas substitution by negatively loaded groups and esterification

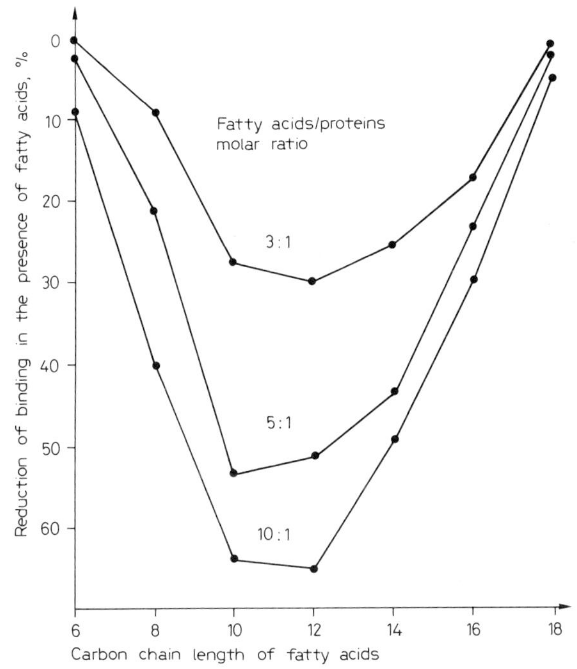

Fig. 4. Influence of fatty acid chain length and concentration on cefazolin binding [according to ref. 6].

cancel it. The fatty acids-human albumin binding would therefore result from hydrophobic interactions rather than from electrostatic or hydrogen bonds.

In vivo Studies

Since the early development of pharmacokinetics and its individualization as an autonomous discipline, many studies have been carried out on the in vivo behavior of drugs from various chemical and pharmacological classes. Only very few of them, however, seem to stress the incidence of FFA levels on protein binding: this possible incidence is either overlooked or considered but then discarded or retained sometimes without experimental data supporting the final conclusion. In the defence of the authors, the intricacy of the mechanisms contributing in vivo to the distribution and the metabolism of drugs complicates seriously these problems, more particularly as these mechanisms vary according to the physicochemical properties of the molecules. Only some studies will be reviewed here.

An interesting in vivo study on diurnal variations of aminophenazone binding according to meal times was recently performed by the equilibrium dialysis method using radiolabeled aminophenazone [13]. Significant differences were found in the percentages of binding according to the nutritional state. In one case, binding averaged 29.8% at 8 a.m. after a 12-hour night fast and 23.3% at 8 p.m. after ingestion of food at 5 p.m., that is a decrease of 22% from 8 a.m. to 8 p.m. under usual dietary conditions. In another case, the amount of binding was 38.1% at 8 a.m. after a 32-hour fast and 32.9% at 8 p.m. after a 44-hour fast, that is a reduction by 14% from 8 a.m. to 8 p.m. The amount of binding in a third case reached 24.8% at 8 a.m. following food intake at 5 a.m. and 31.3% at 8 p.m. after a 12-hour fast, i.e. an increase of 26% from 8 a.m. to 8 p.m. A pharmacokinetic study was carried out in parallel and the results interpreted thanks to those obtained in the work on binding. Food lipids released after meals were thought to displace aminophenazone from its albumin binding sites, thus increasing the proportion of drug available in the free form, ensuring its diffusion in the tissues and consequently increasing the apparent volume of distribution. However, this explanation does not take into account the release of fatty acids under fasting conditions mentioned above. But the release of FFA subsequent to the ingestion of food and that resulting from lipolysis under fasting conditions are very different processes in their intensity and rate which are likely to be higher in the first case.

The other studies which will be reported here are related to diazepam and warfarin which are both highly albumin-bound. It was shown in vitro that adding palmitic and oleic acids so as to obtain a FFA/albumin molar ratio equal to 3 increases the free fraction of diazepam but decreases that of warfarin [10]. Significant variations were also observed in vivo in the same study 2 h after food intake. But inversely the free fraction of diazepam was reduced and that of warfarin increased. The difference in the behavior of the two drugs was assumed to be due to the fact that they bind to two different sites. The decrease in the free fraction following meals was confirmed for diazepam [4] but, however, a previous study had shown no significant change in the binding percentage of this drug under the influence of food [3]. A displacement of the bound fraction of warfarin had been previously observed in rats as soon as the FFA/albumin molar ratio reached 2 [2].

General Interpretation of the Results. Mechanisms of FFA and Drug Bindings [14]. All the results mentioned above show that FFA inhibit plasma albumin binding of drugs or displace them when they are bound. A phenomenon of competition does exist between FFA and drugs for the occupation of the albumin sites. However, the results can be divided into two groups: in one group, FFA have no effect on drug binding as long as their molar concentration is not 2 or 3 times higher than that of albumin; in the other group, FFA intervene at the lowest concentrations and obviously their influence increases more and more.

The variety of the analytical methods used in these studies and their differences in sensitivity may partly explain these two contrary conclusions. The variety of the operating conditions is also likely to be taken into account: the studies are performed either with albumin or serum on the one hand, or with fatty acids used individually which do not necessarily reflect the composition of FFA in vivo on the other hand. Moreover, in vivo studies carried out in a number of animal species bring up the problem about the validity of their extrapolation to other species. Finally all the drugs do not bind in the same way nor on the same sites. Under these conditions, there is a priori no reason for FFA to interfere according to the same mechanisms. These few remarks are sufficient to accept if not to explain in detail the different results obtained.

The interpretation of these results will be now developed. First the absence of interference is admitted at low FFA concentrations but this interpretation can be then extended to such low concentrations. The phenomenon of competition being admitted beyond any consideration of concentration, it is not easy to explain why such a competition does not continue as long as FFA molecules are available if *all* the sites are involved in the competition. If indeed there is no interference of FFA at values of the FFA/albumin molar ratio below 2, it is probably because the albumin molecule can bind to up to 2 mol of FFA without consequence on its drug-binding capacity. This suggests that the albumin molecule has at least two categories of FFA binding sites.

The N_1 sites are really specific of the long-chained FFA which are the only molecules able to penetrate into them either because of their high energy of binding or their long straight chain: drug molecules are unable of binding to those sites because of their weaker energy or their bulky structure. As no displacement is observed below 2 mol of FFA for 1 mol of albumin, the number of N_1 sites with a strong affinity for fatty acids is at least equal to 2/mol of albumin.

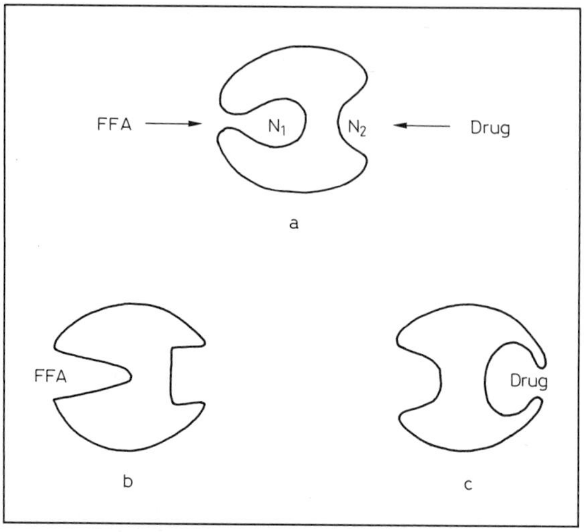

Fig. 5. Schematic illustration of albumin binding of fatty acids and drugs according to the conformational conception [according to ref. 14]: *a* initial conformation before any binding, *b* conformation of N_2 sites altered after the binding of FFA, *c* conformation of N_1 sites altered after the binding of drugs.

The other sites N_2 can bind both FFA and drugs. When the FFA concentration becomes high, the N_1 sites are insufficient to bind them. There is then competition for the occupation of the N_2 sites. There are 4–5 N_2 sites per mol of albumin. One of them was determined to have the only tryptophan residue of the human albumin molecule.

Such a concept of a model where the sites are separate, with some of them being specific for FFA, may be extended so as to become consistent with the results showing a competition even at low FFA concentrations. Conformational changes and/or an extension of the concept of competition may actually account for these results.

First of all one can imagine that the binding of FFA to the N_1 sites induces a change in the 3-dimensional structure of the N_2 sites. This is illustrated schematically in figures 5a and b. The importance of the conformational change might depend on the amount of bound FFA. This would explain the decrease in absorption at 480 nm observed with HABA when the palmitate/albumin molar ratio rises from 0 to 2. Moreover, the conformational change might bring about a progressive variation in the binding strength: the shift of absorption peak towards the longest but less energetic wavelengths observed as the amount of FFA increases would then result from the fact that the molecular interaction between the site and bound HABA varies progressively. However, the assumed conformational change would consist of only minor alterations in the area of the N_2 sites with no considerable change in the tertiary structure of the protein.

Inversely it may be reasonably assumed that the occupation of the N_2 sites by an organic molecule may result in a conformational change in the N_1 sites (fig. 5c). This would explain that clofibrate may displace FFA although it is less strongly bound than them: indeed this phenomenon could be observed.

Another interpretation for the inhibitions or the displacements observed at low FFA amounts may be found in a larger application of the concept of competition. Up to now it has been assumed that FFA would bind to the drug binding sites only when the ratio of their concentration and that of albumin exceeded 2 (considering that the number of sites specific of FFA is 2/mol of albumin). Actually, it is possible to calculate on the basis of the FFA successive association constants (table I) the percentage of albumin molecules which bind 0, 1, 2, 3, ... *n* mol of FFA at given FFA and albumin concentrations. It is thus determined, for instance, that for 2 mol of oleate and 1 mol of albumin, only 40% of the albumin molecules bind to 2 mol of FFA: indeed 6% bind to no mole of FFA, 26% to 1 mol, 20% to 3 mol, 7% to 4 mol and 1% to 5 mol. In other words 28% of the albumin molecules bind to more than 2 mol FFA when FFA/albumin molar ratio is equal to 2. The hypothesis according to which all the drug-binding sites would remain free as long as the molar ratio is below 2 seems therefore inexact. All FFA are not gathered on the only sites which are specific for them, since the difference between the successive association constants (table I) is too low to prevent the occupation of other sites on the same molecule after occupation of the first two. The albumin molecules which have bound to more than 2 mol of FFA have at least some of their drug-binding sites penetrated by FFA. In such an interpretation, competitive phenomena are present even when the molar ratio is below 2. A diminution of the binding strength of drugs results from it which accounts for the decrease ranging from 5 to 15% in the binding observed at FFA/albumin molar ratios between 0 and 2. The shift of the absorption peak of HABA may then likewise be explained by interactions between this compound and the long chains of FFA bound to the drug sites. As compared with the previous one, this second interpretation explains the displacement of drugs via a single mechanism independently of the amount of FFA involved. The phenomenon is simply more intense as the FFA amount increases. Nevertheless, the two processes might intervene simultaneously for the same drug or, on the contrary, different drugs might involve a mechanism which would not be single. Whatever the mechanism(s) involved, it seems that minor increases in the FFA/albumin molar ratio such as those induced by changes in the nutritional state may result in low decreases ranging from 5 to 15% in drug binding, at least for some of them.

What is to be thought of the increased fluorescence observed in the case of ANS on human albumin in the presence of low FFA amounts? This result suggests that low amounts of FFA do not displace ANS but can increase its binding by approximately 10%. The data mentioned above on warfarin substantiate the present conclusion which initially remained isolated. In the study on warfarin, the free fraction decreased under the influence of small FFA amounts [10]. These results tend at least to confirm that small variations in the FFA circulating level within the limits of normal variations are sufficient to influence in one way or in another the binding of the other organic molecules.

Conclusions and Future Prospects

Nutrition may interfere with the plasma binding of drugs according to two pathways which were unequally investigated and whose interest is unequal in wealthy countries. The first pathway is the decrease in plasma albumin levels likely to result in an increased free fraction of the drug because of the deficiency in binding proteins. The second pathway lies in the inhibition of drug binding or in their displacement if they are already bound by substances with a stronger affinity for the binding molecules. In the present work, only the interference of FFA was studied. However, other molecules of endogenous origin can also bind to albumin, thus competing with drugs for the occupation of common sites. Among the molecules likely to depend on nutrition, there are amino acids, in particular tryptophan, which is thought to bind to the same site as a number of drugs do. It may be a priori hypothesized that tryptophan gives rise to interferences of the same nature as FFA. This point should be checked experimentally, as it does not seem to have been investigated up to now. The objection may be raised that the binding site of tryptophan being also a binding site of fatty acids, the latter prevent it from competing since they are themselves competitors.

Another point which should be elucidated is the pharmacological incidence that may cause alterations in binding ranging from 5 to 15% such as those resulting from variations in the FFA circulating level with respect to the nutritional state. Such studies would be particularly relevant with drugs presenting a strong percentage of binding. However, concerning moderately bound drugs whose toxic doses are very close to the efficient doses (for instance methotrexate with an albumin binding averaging 50%), low variations in the percentage of binding might generate unwanted pharmacological and clinical consequences.

The in vitro results should be compared with the in vivo study in man because of the structural differences of albumin in various animal species. Such studies are not difficult to carry out but to interpret. It is clear that many factors are involved in vivo in the metabolism of drugs and in the intensity of the pharmacological effects observed. The plasma binding of drugs should be granted its real place within pharmacokinetic characteristics. These few remarks seem to show that further researches must still be conducted in this field.

References

In view of the long list of studies reviewed in the present work, the bibliography will be restricted to recent studies and to a few reviews of synthesis [5, 11, 14, 15, 17] referring to previous works.

1 Boxer, G.E.; Jelinek, V.C.; Edison, A.O.: Streptomycin. Clearance and binding to protein. J. Pharmac. exp. Ther. *92:* 93–104 (1949).

2 Gugler, R.; Shoeman, D.W.; Azarnoff, D.L.: Effect of in vivo elevation of free fatty acids on protein binding of drugs. Pharmacology *12:* 160–165 (1974).

3 Klotz, U.; Antonin, K.H.; Bieck, P.: Food intake and plasma binding of diazepam. Br. J. clin. Pharmacol. *4:* 85–86 (1977).

4 Naranjo, C.A.; Sellers, E.M.; Giles, H.G.; Abel, J.G.: Diurnal variations in plasma diazepam concentrations associated with reciprocal changes in free fraction. Br. J. clin. Pharmacol. *9:* 265–272 (1980).

5 Peters, T., Jr.: Serum albumin; in Putnam, The plasma proteins; 2nd ed., pp. 133–181 (Academic Press, New York 1975).

6 Pitkin, D.H.; Actor, P.; Weisbach, J.A.: Serum protein binding alterations of selected cephalosporin antibiotics by fatty acids and their derivatives. J. pharm. Sci. *69:* 354–356 (1980).

7 Prasad, J.S.; Krishnaswamy, K.: Streptomycin pharmacokinetics in malnutrition. Chemotherapy *24:* 333–337 (1978).

8 Raghuram, T.C.; Krishnaswamy, K.: Tetracycline kinetics in undernourished subjects. Int. J. clin. Pharm. Ther. Tox. *19:* 409–413 (1981).

9 Rowell, F.J.; Hui, S.M.; Fairbairn, A.F.; Eccleston, D.: Total and free serum haloperidol levels in schizophrenic patients and the effect of age, thioridazine and fatty acid on haloperidol-serum protein binding in vitro. Br. J. clin. Pharmacol. *11:* 377–382 (1981).
10 Sellers, E.M.; Naranjo, C.A.; Abel, J.G.; Khouw, V.; Sandor, P.; Alexander, P.: Fatty acid (FA) modulation of reciprocal variation in diazepam (Dα) and warfarin free fraction (Wα) (résumé). Clin. Pharmacol. Ther. *27:* 285–286 (1980).
11 Settle, W.; Hegeman, S.; Featherstone, R.M.: The nature of drug-protein interaction; in Brodie, Gillette, Concepts in biochemical pharmacology, part 1, pp. 175–186 (Springer, Berlin 1971).
12 Shastri, A.R.; Krishnaswamy, K.: Undernutrition and tetracycline half-life. Clinica chim. Acta *66:* 157–164 (1976).
13 Shively, C.A.; Simons, R.J.; Passananti, G.T.; Dvorchik, B.H.; Vesell, E.S.: Dietary patterns and diurnal variations in aminopyrine disposition. Clin. Pharmacol. Ther. *29:* 65–73 (1981).
14 Spector, A.A.; Fletcher, J.E.: Nutritional effects on drug-protein binding; in Hathcock, Coon, Nutrition and drug interrelations, pp. 447–473 (Academic Press, New York 1978).
15 Tillement, J.P.: Fixation des médicaments sur les protéines plasmatiques; in Giroud, Mathé, Mayniel, Pharmacologie clinique. Bases de la thérapeutique, I, pp. 151–164 (Expansion scientifique française, Paris 1978).
16 Urien, S.; Albengres, E.; Tillement, J.P.: Serum protein binding of valproic acid in healthy subjects and in patients with liver disease. Int. J. clin. Pharm. Ther. Tox. *19:* 319–325 (1981).
17 Vallner, J.J.: Binding of drugs by albumin and plasma protein. J. pharm. Sci. *66:* 447–465 (1977).

A. Gayte-Sorbier, MD, Laboratoire de Bromatologie, Diététique et Analyse appliquée à l'Expertise, Faculté de Pharmacie, 27, boulevard Jean-Moulin, F-13385 Marseille Cedex 5 (France)

Wld Rev. Nutr. Diet., vol. 43, pp. 117–128 (Karger, Basel 1984)

Food and Drug Interactions

R.J. Royer[a], *G. Debry*[b], *M. Ulmer*[b], *B. Bannwarth*[a]

[a]Centre Hospitalier Régional de Nancy, Laboratoire de Pharmacologie;
[b]Département de Nutrition et des Maladies Métaboliques de l'Université de Nancy, Unité de Recherches de Nutrition et de Diététique de l'INSERM, U. 59, Nancy, France

Introduction

It is not unexpected that drugs, such as for instance xenobiotics, show interactions with the various chemicals present in our natural or induced environment. Food and drug chemical interactions, adsorptions, chelations, direct or indirect transformations are not infrequent in the alimentary canal. Food, by altering the rate of the passage or the concentration of drugs, generates changes in the absorption conditions. Digestive absorption also depends on two elements present simultaneously.

Metabolisms, in particular the liver metabolism, are interdependent. Some elements absorbed may mutually alter their toxicity. Elimination also depends on various factors, such as pH, which can be modified by either substance present. Bioavailability, which is the aggregate expression of the above elements, is frequently deeply influenced. Malabsorptions or neutralizations, particularly of vitamins, are occasionally observed.

The aim of the present work is not to review these points systematically. Some of them have been developed in other parts of this work. Particular attention will be paid to some special aspects of food and drug interactions.

Local Interactions in the Digestive Tract

Rate of the Passage [2, 59]

At the Level of the Stomach

The alimentary bolus first stops in the stomach which is normally emptied exponentially [31]. The volume of the stomach, water, the low temperature of food [62] and the low osmotic power [30] accelerate gastric emptying.

Some drugs, such as anticholinergics, psycholeptics, antacids, analgesics, and narcotic analgesics, may delay the digestive passage. Fats, in particular long-chained lipids [31, 32], unsaturated triglycerides [68], carbohydrates, and proteins at high concentrations [11, 29] also slow gastric emptying.

The incidence of slowing at this level is particularly discernible for drugs. – Alkaloids, substances destroyed by hydrolysis, do not stand a prolonged stay in the stomach. – Drugs not absorbed at the gastric level have a delayed kinetics of absorption. – Drugs crossing the gastric membrane are, however, little influenced (aspirin and weak acids generally). – Some weak bases are better transformed into salts which are more easily assimilable by the upper parts of the alimentary canal.

At the Gut Level

The gut is the major site of absorption due to the large surface developed by villositis and due to the peristaltis-related regular mixing. However, when peristaltis is too important, substances in the gut remain for a lesser time and sustained-release products are not completely resorbed. So it is with substances having specific absorption areas (vitamin B_1, vitamin B_{12}). Food is the natural stimulant of the passage. Due to its composition, it is capable of altering the secretions and the digestive flora and even involves unwanted motor reactions of the alimentary canal.

Dilution of Drugs and Food [61]

The water absorbed passes rapidly through the stomach into the system in which it induces a light dilution of plasma before it is eliminated by the kidneys. Dilution should facilitate the absorption of water-soluble drugs and affect liposoluble drugs unfavorably.

Actually, the notion of dilution is controversial. *Ferguson* [19] has shown that many substances, such as pentobarbital or aspirin, were better absorbed with increasing dilution. These solutions are hypotonic and present a larger volume distributed over a larger intestinal surface [6].

Dissolution of Drugs

– Drugs are mostly absorbed in the solid form and ought to be above all solubilized. Carbohydrates may enhance this dissolution. Sugars have been suspected of increasing the solubilization of bismuth subnitrate or a number of heavy metals. The solubility of bismuth salts is also enhanced by polyols, such as sorbitol, tartric acid, and gluconic acid [58]. In the presence of vinegar, its solubility is far from negligible [25]. The absorption of acids, alcohol, and bases may enhance or delay the dissolution of the drug according to its nature.

– Fat intake induces a strong secretion of acids and bile salts which are surface-active agents enhancing dissolution in the gut [4] of phenolphthalein [57], phenytoin [50], carbamazepine [46] and griseofulvin [4, 12, 37].

– Excess viscosity of the alimentary bolus may slow the bioavailability of propranolol [49]. Proteins act frequently as enhancing agents of viscosity but natural mucin may be also implicated. Irritating substances may produce it in excess. This was shown for tetracycline [65].

– Some drugs – almost insoluble in water, such as griseofulvin – may be more easily solubilized if taken with fat food, thus being better absorbed [12, 13].

Solubilization of course depends on the pH of the medium, and any change in pH attributable to food or drugs ought to be taken into consideration. Acid drugs are less soluble in an acid medium and basic drugs at high pH. The factor 'dissolution' is worth investigation. Today Galenic researchers use all these data in support of the most efficient formulation possible for a given situation.

Antacids and Covering Agents

Only non-systemic antacids with an essentially local digestive action will be reviewed in the present work. Although they are not considered as food they are so much involved in the digestive comfort that they cannot be ignored. Compounds ensuring interaction with drugs are primarily aluminum and magnesium salts. Owing to their neutralizing power, they intervene at all stages of dissolution, transformation and absorption of drugs.

From all studies conducted, there emerges a reduction of absorption for acid drugs in general, and in particular for furosemide, tetracyclines, digoxin, isoniazids, anticholinergics, and indomethacin [23, 69] by aluminum salts. They have no effect on amoxicillin, troleandomycin (TAO), prednisone or ketoprofen [23, 69]. Their incidence in nutrition is still unclear.

Direct Chemical Interactions

Food and drugs may chelate, neutralize reciprocally, form insoluble complexes and precipitate.

– Penicillin loses part of its activity if it is absorbed after fat intake. Its persistence in the stomach thus enhanced ensures the opening of the β-lactame cycle thus making it inactive [26, 35].

– Tetracycline forms a non-absorbed complex in the presence of proteins [36], magnesium [15], calcium in milk food [38], and iron in some food [24, 55]. The elements of the complex ought to be administered simultaneously. In the presence of tripalmitine eliminating calcium ions, tetracycline is much more active than when administered conventionally.

– Heavy metal ions and various macromolecules are also capable of chelating this antibiotic [71]. Doxycycline is much less affected. These effects disappear if a few hours' interval separates the administration of the drug and that of food.

– The interrelation between food rich in tannin, such as strong tea, coffee, quince, some wines, etc., and drugs or some metals is less clear. Tannins form a complex with iron and the other heavy metals which are then no longer reabsorbed. Tea is also capable of capturing iron present in food, such as rice, potatoes, bread, and walnuts, thus depriving them from part of their nutritive properties [3]. In strict vegetarian diets, tea and water are generally the basic drinks. This explains pathologies related to an iron deficiency. Tea and coffee are capable of neutralizing many alkaloids. For that reason, administration of very strong tea is recommended in the case of intoxication by alkaloids or heavy metals. Tea and coffee are also capable of precipitating phenothiazines [8].

– Another example of interaction is found in the formation of complexes between iron, various important oligoelements, such as cobalt, manganese and zinc on the one hand, and polyuronides, such as pectins and alginates, on the other hand. These substances are largely used in the industrial preparation of soups, jams, ready-cooked sweets, etc. Severe dysfunctions, which are generally ill-characterized clinically, may appear in the case of regular and prolonged use of these products.

– Mucin, a natural mucopolysaccharide, may chelate some active principles, such as streptomycines, anticholinergics, antihypertensive agents, etc. Food and drugs, in particular antiinflammatory agents which alter the content or the composition of mucin, may generate interaction. Interestingly, chelation by calcium or aluminum ions, of caffein or ergotamine, enhances the absorption of these products [23].

These examples are not infrequent and interactions with cholestyramine may be connected with them. Further studies will undoubtedly clear up some aspects of drug and food cohabitation which are still unexplained.

Drugs Modified by Enzymes and the Digestive Flora

The role of gastric juice is to digest food. Some drugs may behave as enzyme inhibitors (disulfiram, highly oxidating or reducing products) and enzymes as substances altering drugs by deacetylation, hydrolysis of esters by non-specific esterases or lipases [1, 22].

The influence of the digestive flora, either normal or modified by dietary regimen, has been studied in the animal model [60] but not really confirmed in man. Again, reactions of hydrolysis, reduction, degradation into compounds of lower molecular weight, decarboxylations, dealkylation, dehalogenation, deamination, esterification, acetylation, etc. Drugs may produce, in the case of infections or intestinal microbial pathologies, unexpected metabolites. The pharmacological action of these metabolites may prove particular.

Overall Pharmacokinetic Aspect

Phenomena of local interactions in the alimentary canal are worth attention more particularly as they may occur in an opposite direction during digestive absorption or the later stages. Illustrative of such are basic drugs. Tablets of these drugs are more soluble in acid medium but their important ionization makes gastric absorption difficult. A few examples of aggregate drug and food interactions will be referred to [48, 70].

It has been shown in man that the composition and the volume of drinks did not alter warfarin absorption. Food does not really affect the bioavailability of the product. However, a large consumption of vegetables, such as spinach or cabbage, rich in vitamin K, enhances prothrombinemia in patients on anticoagulant therapy.

An alkaline diet associated with cow's milk and vitamin D in normal quantities induced an idiopathic hypercalcemia in infants [59]. The absorption of sulfonamide, 5-methoxy-sulfadiazine, was enhanced when administered with a lipid-enriched meal as compared to a protein or carbohydrate diet [33]. Much remains to be explained in this field.

A Few Special Interactions

One of the best-known interactions is that between monoamine oxidase (MAO) inhibitors and some food [16, 59]. The drugs concerned are antidepressants, such as iproniazid, tranylcypromine, pargyline or phenelzine, and food that contains tyramine or other sympathomimetic amines or their precursors. Some cheeses, yeasts, yoghourts, beers or wines, such as Chianti or port, are known to induce hypertensive attacks which are sometimes fatal. Broad beans, which contain 3,4-dihydroxyphenylalanine (DOPA) have identical effects [5, 28].

Hypokalemia induced by glycyrrhizin, found in drinks and licorice confectionery, may generate disorders in the heart rate in cases of concomitant digitoxin treatment. Renal dysfunction, myopathies, and myoglobinuria may appear more particularly if hypokalemic diuretics are given in addition.

Glutamates used in Chinese food, in particular Won ton, a popular soup, may give rise to a syndrome characterized by headaches, sensations of burn in the extremities, thoracic pains and hot flushes. This syndrome is probably related to hyponatremia. Diuretics may be a triggering or aggravating factor [59, 66]. Some goitrogenic food, such as Brussels sprouts, Swedish turnips, turnips, and cauliflower, may potentiate synthetic antithyroid drugs [39].

Alcohol and disulfiram (Antabuse) induce a characteristic flush. Many drugs (metronidazole and antidiabetic sulfonamides) have similar properties. Drug-related allergic reactions are observed after sensitization by food containing these materials (antibiotics and hormones).

Hyperglycemia may be induced by nicotinic acid present in some food to prevent it from going black. In diabetic subjects, this effect may hinder considerably the therapeutic equilibrium [52].

Drug-Alcohol Interaction

This interaction is justified in the present work if alcohol is considered as food. This problem will not be reviewed exhaustively as the literature is not sparse with works on this subject. Again, only a few illustrations will be referred to [53, 56, 64]. Ethanol is a factor of digestive disturbance. Used chronically, it may result in malabsorptions [53], in particular those of xylose, methionine and vitamin A which have been demonstrated.

Drug action is appreciably altered in chronic alcoholics only at the final stage of cirrhosis. On the other hand, in acute administration, alcohol through its vasodilating action accelerates the phenomenon of absorption. Alcohol potentiates the sensitivity of receptors to psychotropic drugs. Alcohol is capable of altering the metabolism and degradation conditions of phenobarbital, meprobamate, diphenylhydantoin, antipyrine, and tolbutamide by stimulating the microsomal system. It inhibits, however, the transformation of hexobarbital via an indirect phenomenon, thus inducing a hypersecretion of glucocorticoids.

Inversely, drugs may interfere with the metabolism of alcohol. Neuroleptics, such as chlorpromazine and chloral, inhibit dehydrogenase and enhance alcoholemia. Disulfiram, griseofulvin, hypoglycemic sulfonamides, phenacetin, and MAO inhibitors inhibit dehydrogenase acetaldehyde and increse the toxicity of alcohol. This drug and alcohol interaction is multiform and probably one of the most relevant problems when one knows its incidence on road or labor safety.

Toxicity of Drug and Food Association

Food Nitrates

These originate in largely used fertilizers. Carrots and spinach in particular contain a high percentage of food nitrates [47, 67]. Nitrates on their own are not very toxic but they may turn into nitrites under the influence of bacteria or more simply when vegetables are not fresh or are warmed-up. The production of methemoglobin is a well-known phenomenon in young children whose blood contains a high proportion of fetal hemoglobin [27].

In an acid-digestive medium, nitrates may combine with secondary amines to form nitrosamines, the carcinogenic action of which has been well-established. These amines are largely present in food and the reaction is most frequent (walnuts, tomatoes, bananas) [14, 18, 20]. Secondary or tertiary amines may also originate in drugs; for instance amidopyrine, or aminophenazone, is particularly reactive. Actually, it is gradually being withdrawn from the market [3]. Ephedrine and anorexant amines may also intervene. Anthelmintics and piperazine derivatives lead to the formation of dinitrosopiperazine which is also a carcinogenic compound [3].

Nitrites combine with ascorbic acid, thus giving nitrates, nitrogen oxide, and dehydroascorbic acid [3]. It might be considered that this action causes a vitamin C deficiency or that ascorbic acid can be used to neutralize excess nitrites.

Carbon Tetrachloride

This chemical is used in certain industries. It is absorbed by the workers exposed to it. Although it is not a drug, it is closely related to drugs due to its permanent presence in the system. Actually, there exists a toxic effect after transformation by cytochrome P-450 of the microsomal system. A protein-poor diet reduces the enzyme activity and decreases the toxicity of carbon tetrachloride [21, 43, 44].

Aflatoxins

Inversely, the carcinogenic effects of aflatoxins are blocked by the drugs inducing the activity of cytochrome P-450 (phenobarbital, rifampicinum, etc.). It would be a complex effect ensuring the neutralization of reactive epoxy by concomitant stimulation of hydratase epoxy.

Paracetamol

The liver toxicity of this drug is observed at the level of cytochrome P-450 by formation of reactive metabolites which react by combining preferentially with glutathione. When the glutathione level falls below 1 m*M*, these metabolites combine with the macromolecules and bring about toxic phenomena [51]. A protein-rich diet enhances toxicity while a protein-poor diet reduces it [40, 42, 72]. The origins of these effects are complex. Other diets are also capable of modifying the toxicity of paracetamol [41].

Conclusions

In the present work particular attention is paid to the large variety of food and drug interactions. The specific mechanisms which contribute to the analysis and understanding of the different modes of action are not reviewed in detail. Other parts in this work are more detailed. It is evident that the very large number of drugs available to us and the diversity of the food we absorb require considerable efforts of research.

References

1 Agersborg, H.P.; Batchelor, A.; Cambridge, G.W.; Rule, A.W.: The pharmacology of penamecillin. Br. J. Pharmacol. *26:* 649–655 (1966).

2 Aiache, J.M.: Influence des régimes alimentaires sur l'absorption des médicaments. Pharm. Acta Helv. *55:* 210–220 (1980).

3 Becker, G.: Nahrungsmittel als Störfaktoren in der Pharmacotherapie. Medsche Welt, Stuttg. *29:* 1163–1166 (1978).

4 Bedford, C.; Bushfield, D.; Child, K.J.; MacGregor, I.; Sutherland, P.; Tomich, E.G.: Studies on the biological disposition of griseofulvin, an oral antifungal agent. Archs Derm. *81:* 735–745 (1960).

5 Beneton, C.: Tyramine: aliments et vin. Bulletin d'information du médicament. Pharmacovigilance, No. 10, pp. 11–12 (CHR, Rennes 1981).

6 Borowitz, J.L.; Moore, P.F.; Yim, G.K.M.; Miya, T.S.: Mechanism of enhanced drug effects produced by dilution of the oral dose. Toxicol. appl. Pharmacol. *19:* 164–168 (1971).

7 Carr, C.J.: Food and drug interactions. Annu. Rev. Pharmacol. Toxicol. *22:* 19–29 (1982).

8 Cheeseman, H.J.; Neal, M.J.: Interaction of chlorpromazine with tea and coffee. Br. J. clin. Pharmac. *12:* 165–169 (1981).

9 Conney, A.H.; Pantuck, E.J.; Kuntzman, R.; Kappas, A.; Anderson, K.E.; Alvares, A.P.: Nutrition and chemical biotransformations in man. Clin. Pharmacol. Ther. *22:* 707–720 (1977).

10 Conney, A.H.; Pantuck, E.J.; Hsiao, K.C.; Kuntzman, R.; Alvares, A.P.; Kappas, A.: Regulation of drug metabolism in man by environmental chemicals and diet. Fed. Proc. *36:* 1647–1652 (1977).

11 Cooke, A.R.; Moulang, J.: Control of gastric emptying by amino-acids. Gastroenterology *62:* 528–532 (1972).

12 Crounse, R.G.: Human pharmacology of griseofulvin: the effect of fat intake on gastrointestinal absorption. J. invest. Derm. *37:* 529–533 (1961).

13 Crounse, R.G.: Effective use of griseofulvin. Archs Derm. *87:* 176–178 (1963).

14 Crout, J.P.; Sjoerdsma, A.: The clinical and laboratory significance of serotonin and catecholamines in bananas. New Engl. J. Med. *261:* 23–26 (1959).

15 Dearborn, E.H.; Lichtfield, J.T., Jr.; Eisner, H.J.; Corbett, J.J.; Dunett, C.W.: The effects of various substances on the absorption of tetracycline in rats. Antibiotic Med. clin. Ther. *4:* 627–641 (1957).

16 Dickerson, J.W.T.: Some adverse effects of drugs on nutrition. R. Soc. Hlth J. *98:* 261–265 (1978).

17 Descotes, J.; Rotivel, Y.; Loupi, E.: Médicaments et alimentation. Conséquences pharmacologiques et effets indésirables. Lyon Pharm. *31:* 239–240 (1980).

18 Editorial: Fd Cosmet. Toxicol. *2:* 228 (1964).

19 Ferguson, H.C.: Dilution of dose and oral toxicity. Toxicol. appl. Pharmacol. *4:* 759–762 (1962).

20 Foy, J.M.; Parrat, J.R.: A note on the presence of noradrenaline and 5-hydroxytryptamine in plantain *(Musa sapientum,* var. *paradisiaca).* J. Pharm. Pharmacol. *12:* 360–364 (1960).

21 Garner, R.C.; McLean, A.E.M.: Increased susceptibility to carbon tetrachloride poisoning in the rat after pretreatment with oral phenobarbitone. Biochem. Pharmacol. *18:* 645–650 (1969).

22 Glazko, A.J.; Edgerton, W.H.; Dill, W.A.; Lenz, W.R.: Chloromycetin palmitate – synthetic ester of chloromycetin. Antibiotics Chemother. *2:* 234–242 (1952).

23 Goodman, L.S.; Gilman, A.: The pharmacological basis of therapeutics; 5th ed. (Macmillan, New York 1975).

24 Gothoni, G.; Neuvonen, P.J.; Mattila, M.; Hackman, R.: Iron-tetracycline interaction: effect of time interval between the drugs. Acta med. scand. *191:* 409–411 (1972).

25 Goulle, J.P.: Spectrophotométrie d'absorption atomique. Détection de traces de Cd, Cu, Pb, Zn dans les additifs aux médicaments et aliments; étude de la solubilité des chélates de bismuth; thèse, Rouen (1975).

26 Heatley, N.G.: Comparative serum concentration and excretion experiments with benzyl penicillin (G) and phenoxymethyl penicillin (V) on single subject. Antibiotic Med. *2:* 33–41 (1956).

27 Holscher, P.M.; Natzschka, J.: Methämoglobinämie bei jungen Säuglingen durch nitrithaltigen Spinat. Dt. med. Wschr. *89:* 1751–1754 (1964).

28 Horwitz, D.; Lovenberg, W.; Engelman, K.; Sjoerdsma, A.: Monoamine oxidase inhibitors, tyramine and cheese. J. Am. med. Ass. *188:* 1108–1110 (1964).

29 Hunt, J.N.; Pathak, J.D.: The osmotic effects of some simple molecules and ions on gastric emptying. J. Physiol., Lond. *154:* 254–269 (1960).

30 Hunt, J.N.; Knox, M.T.: Control of gastric emptying. Am. J. dig. Dis. *13:* 372–388 (1968).

31 Hunt, J.N.; Knox, M.T.: Regulation of gastric emptying. Handbook of Physiology, sect. 6, vol. 4, pp. 1917–1935 (Am. Physiological Society, Washington 1968).

32 Hunt, J.N.; Knox, M.T.: A relation between the chain length of fatty acids and the slowing of gastric emptying. J. Physiol., Lond. *194:* 327–336 (1968).

33 Kaumeier, S.: The effect of the composition of food on the absorption of sulfameter. Int. J. clin. Pharmacol. Biopharm. *17:* 260–263 (1979).

34 Kenny, A.D.: Drugs and nutrition. Fed. Proc. *38:* 2655–2658 (1979).

35 Klein, J.O.; Finland, M.: Ampicillin. Activity in vitro and absorption and excretion in normal young men. Am. J. med. Sci. *245:* 544–555 (1963).

36 Kohn, K.W.: Mediation of divalent metal ions in the binding of tetracycline to macromolecules. Nature, Lond. *191:* 1156–1158 (1961).

37 Kraml, M.; Dubuc, J.; Beall, D.: Gastrointestinal absorption of griseofulvin. I. Effect of particle size, addition of surfactants and corn oil on the level of griseofulvin in the serum of rats. Can. J. Biochem. *40:* 1449–1451 (1962).

38 Kunin, C.M.; Finland, M.: Clinical pharmacology of the tetracycline antibiotics. Clin. Pharmacol. Ther. *2:* 51–69 (1961).

39 Lamy, P.P.; Blake, D.A.: Therapeutic incompatibilities. J. Am. pharm. Ass. *10:* 72–77 (1970).

40 Leaf, G.; Neuberger, A.: The effect of diet on the glutathione content of the liver. Biochem. J. *41:* 280–287 (1947).

41 McLean, A.E.M.: Diet, DDT, and the toxicity of drugs and chemicals. Fed. Proc. *36:* 1688–1691 (1977).

42 McLean, A.E.M.; Day, P.A.: The effect of diet in the toxicity of paracetamol and the safety of paracetamol methionine mixtures. Biochem. Pharmacol. *24:* 37–42 (1974).

43 McLean, A.E.M.; McLean, E.K.: Diet, microsomal enzymes and CCL_4 toxicity. Biochem. J. *97:* 31 (1965).

44 McLean, A.E.M.; McLean, E.K.: The effect of diet and DDT on microsomal hydroxylating enzymes and on the sensitivity of rats to CCL_4 poisoning. Biochem. J. *100:* 564–571 (1966).

45 McLean, A.E.M.; Marshall, A.K.: The inhibitory effect of phenobarbitone on aflatoxin carcinogenesis. Br. J. exp. Path. *52:* 322–329 (1971).

46 Levy, R.H.; Pitlick, W.H.; Troupin, A.S.; Green, J.R.; Neal, J.M.: Pharmacokinetics of carbamazepine in normal man. Clin. Pharmacol. Ther. *17:* 657–668 (1975).

47 Ludewig, R.; Lohs, K.: Akute Vergiftungen; 4. Aufl., S. 305 (Fischer, Stuttgart 1974).

48 Melander, A.: Influence of food on the bioavailability of drugs. Clin. Pharmacokinet. *3:* 337–351 (1978).

49 Melander, A.; Danielson, K.; Scherstein, B.; Wahlin, E.: Enhancement of the bioavailability of propranolol and metroprolol by food. Clin. Pharmacol. Ther. *22:* 108–112 (1977).

50 Melander, A.; Brante, G.; Johannson, O.; Lindberg, T.; Whalin-Bool, E.: Influence of food intake on the absorption of phenytoin in man. Eur. J. clin. Pharmacol. *15:* 269–274 (1979).

51 Mitchell, J.R.; Jollow, D.J.; Potter, W.Z.: Acetaminophen-induced hepatic necrosis. I. Role of drug metabolism. J. Pharm. exp. Ther. *187:* 185–194 (1973).

52 Molnar, G.D.; Berge, K.G.; Rosevear, J.W.: The effect of nicotinic acid in diabetes mellitus. Metabolism *13:* 181–190 (1964).

53 Morgan, M.Y.: Alcohol and nutrition. Br. med. Bull. *38:* 21–29 (1982).

54 Musa, M.N.; Lyons, L.L.: Absorption and disposition of warfarin: effects of food and liquids. Curr. ther. Res. *20:* 630–633 (1976).

55 Neuvonen, P.J.; Gothoni, G.; Hackman, R.; Bjorksten, K.A.: Interference of iron with the absorption of tetracycline in man. Br. med. J. *iv:* 532–534 (1970).

56 Nordmann, R.: Alcool et médicaments: interférences métaboliques. Revue Alcoolisme *22:* 1–5 (1976).

57 Pekanmaki, K.; Salmi, H.A.: The absorption and excretion of phenolphtalein and its glucuronide by the cat. Acta pharmac. tox. *18:* 133–140 (1961).

58 Pellerin, F.; Goulle, J.P.; Dumitrescu, D.: Formation des chélates solubles de bismuth en présence de divers médicaments et aliments. Revue fr. Gastroent. *128:* 27–41 (1977).

59 Pierpauli, P.G.: Drug therapy and diet. Drug Intell. clin. Pharm. *6:* 89–99 (1972).

60 Prins, R.A.: Nutritional impact of intestinal drug-microbe interaction, pp. 189–251 (Academic Press, New York 1978).

61 Quevauviller, A.: Régime alimentaire et activité des médicaments. Méd. Afr. Noire *21:* 109–117 (1974).

62 Ritschel, W.A.; Erni, W.: The influence of temperature of ingested fluid on stomach emptying time. Int. J. clin. Pharm. Biopharm. *15:* 172–175 (1977).
63 Romankiewicz, J.A.; Reidenberg, M.M.: Factors that modify drug absorption. Ration. Drug Ther. *12:* 1–5 (1978).
64 Royer, R.J.: Interférence des médicaments et de l'alcool. Annls Méd. Nancy *17:* 1115–1118 (1978).
65 Saggers, B.A.; Lawson, D.: Some observations on the penetration of antibiotics through mucus in vitro. J. clin. Path. *19:* 313–317 (1966).
66 Schaumburg, H.H.; Byck, R.; Gerstl, R.; Mashman, J.H.: Monosodium *L*-glutamate: its pharmacology and role in the Chinese restaurant syndrome. Science *163:* 826–828 (1969).
67 Simon, C.: Nitrite poisoning from spinach (letter). Lancet *i:* 872 (1966).
68 Tidwell, H.C.; Cameron, E.S.: Relation between chemical structure of fats and their ability to produce gastric inhibition. Bull. Johns Hopkins Hosp. *70:* 362–369 (1942).
69 Vidal: Dictionnaire (OVP, Paris 1982).
70 Welling, P.G.: Influence of food and diet on gastrointestinal drug absorption: a review. J. Pharmacokinet. Biopharm. *5:* 291–334 (1977).
71 Welling, P.G.: The influence of food on the absorption of antimicrobial agents. J. antimicrob. Chemother. *9:* 7–27 (1982).
72 Woodcock, B.G.; Wood, G.C.: Effect of protein-free diet on UDP-glucuronyltransferase and sulphotransferase activities in rat liver. Biochem. Pharmacol. *20:* 2703–2713 (1971).

R.J. Royer, MD,
Centre Hospitalier Régional de Nancy, Laboratoire de Pharmacologie,
29, avenue du Maréchal-de-Lattre-de-Tassigny,
F–54000 Nancy (France)

Wld Rev. Nutr. Diet., vol. 43, pp. 129–139 (Karger, Basel 1984)

Effect of Protein-Energy Malnutrition on Drug Metabolism in Man[1]

N. Buchanan

Department of Paediatrics, University of Sydney, Westmead Centre, Westmead, Sydney, Australia

Protein energy malnutrition (PEM, previously called protein calorie malnutrition, PCM) is one of the world's greatest health problems – it was conservatively estimated in 1974 that approximately 100,000,000 children aged 0–4 years had moderate to severe PEM [2]. There is no reason to believe that this figure has anything but increased during the intervening years. PEM is subject to a number of classifications, of which the Wellcome classification is perhaps the most widely used (table I) [16]. For those who have not encountered malnourished children, figure 1 shows a child with kwashiorkor and figure 2, a marasmic child. Marasmic kwashiorkor represents a combination of the two, namely marasmus with oedema (fig. 3).

The mortality of hospitalised children with kwashiorkor remains at 20–25% with death being due mainly to overwhelming infection despite the fact that many of these children receive 'appropriate' antimicrobial therapy (e.g. ampicillin, penicillin and kanamycin, etc.). It is this observation which was the starting point for our investigations. Are these children not responding because they present too late for treatment, because they have diminished cell-mediated immunity or because therapy was in fact inappropriate? As there was no way to influence the first two factors, it was decided to concentrate on the third one; was therapy, especially with antimicrobials, as being administered on a standard mg/kg body weight basis, in fact appropriate? Reviewing the pathophysiology of kwashiorkor revealed a number of abnormalities which could alter pharmacokinetics/dynamics in these

[1] Based on work carried out at Baragwanath Hospital, Johannesburg, and supported by the South African Medical Research Council.

1 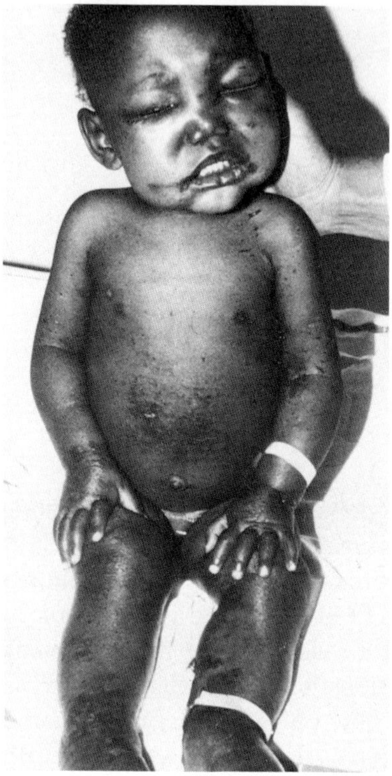

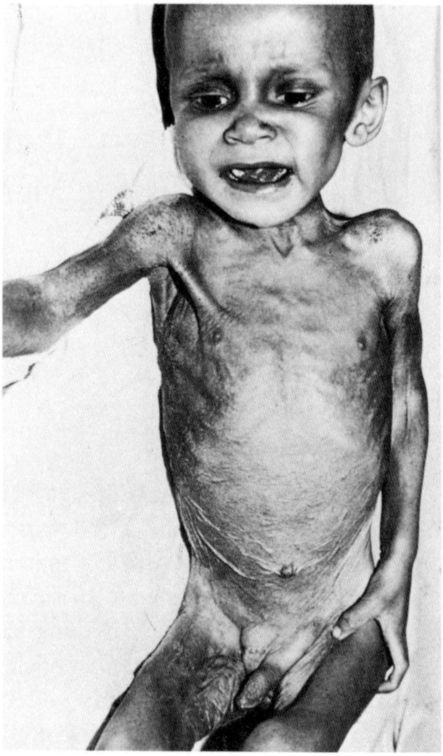 2

Fig. 1. A child with kwashiorkor showing profound oedema.
Fig. 2. A marasmic child showing gross emaciation.

Table I. Wellcome classification of malnutrition

	Body weight as % of standard	Presence of oedema
Underweight child	80–60	–
Marasmus	60	–
Kwashiorkor	80–60	+
Marasmic kwashiorkor	60	+

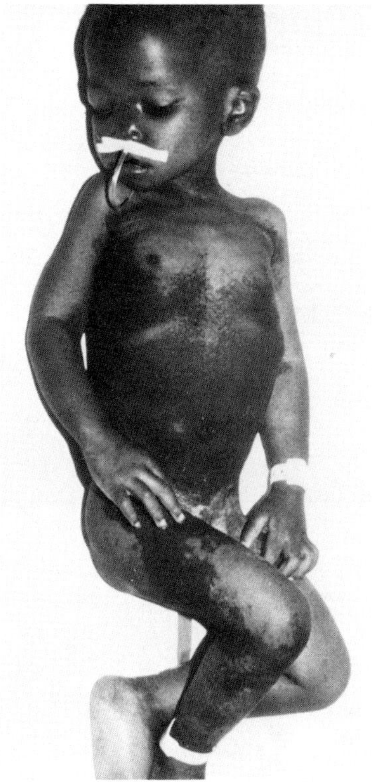

Fig. 3. Marasmic kwashiorkor, showing wasting and oedema.

children (table II). It was especially the abnormalities of renal and hepatic function which it was felt might influence drug disposition in PEM.

This paper attempts to summarise the systematic efforts of our group to look at this problem and to compare our results to those of colleagues in India and South America.

Materials and Methods

These differed slightly for each drug studied; however, certain principles remained unchanged: (a) Informed consent was obtained from parents prior to any studies being performed. (b) Each child acted as their own control, being studied on admission and subsequently 21 days later when nutritionally rehabilitated [6]. (c) Only children with kwashiorkor were studied.

Table II. Pathophysiological changes in PEM which may alter pharmacokinetics

1	*Drug absorption*
	Oedema of limbs relevant to intramuscular absorption
	Mucosal atrophy of bowel
	Rapid intestinal transit (diarrhoea)
2	*Drug distribution*
	Hypoalbuminaemia
	Increased extracellular and total body water
3	*Drug metabolism*
	Abnormal liver functions
	Fatty liver
4	*Drug excretion*
	Decreased renal plasma flow
	Decreased glomerular filtration

Results

Drug Absorption

Intramuscular

As many hospitalised children with PEM receive antibiotics by the intramuscular route (i.m.), it was important to ensure that i.m. bioavailability was acceptable in the presence of gross oedema. This was shown to be the case for penicillin, tobramycin and cefoxitin, except in the presence of absolutely gross oedema (greater than 30% of body weight) [3, 5, 12]. It was thus concluded that, except in the grossly oedematous or shocked child, i.m. antibiotic administration was therapeutically acceptable.

Gastro-Intestinal Absorption

This has been studied essentially with two drugs; tetracyclines and chloramphenicol. Tetracycline bioavailability was shown to be impaired by 50% in undernourished adults [24], but the clinical significance of this observation is uncertain as these findings were unrelated to clinical effect. The data on chloramphenicol is more confusing, as children with PEM were observed to have delayed absorption but higher peak drug levels [20]. It is difficult to reconcile these two observations. The data to hand so far does not suggest that the patient with mild to moderate PEM, who might be treated with oral medication, has a significant absorptive problem.

Drug Distribution

Volume of Distribution

Shastri and Krishnaswamy [25] showed the volume of distribution of tetracycline to be reduced in acute PEM. Our group confirmed this observation with gentamicin [8], cefoxitin [12], isoniazid [7], acetanilide [11] and antipyrine [10]. This would imply higher serum drug concentrations for the same mg/kg dose than in well-nourished individuals.

Plasma Protein Binding

One of the hallmarks of kwashiorkor is hypoalbuminaemia with albumin which is qualitatively normal [23]. *Shastri and Krishnaswamy* [24] have reported diminished tetracycline binding to plasma proteins, whilst *Krishnaswamy* et al. [19] made similar observations with phenylbutazone, as did *Mönckeberg* et al. [21] with salicylates. Our group [4] studied the in vitro binding of 18 drugs to kwashiorkor serum using an equilibrium dialysis technique. Drugs studied included chloramphenicol, penicillin, sulphamethoxazole, gentamicin, cloxacillin, flucloxacillin, streptomycin, ethambutol, ethionamide, isoniazid, para-aminosalicylic acid, rifampicin, phenobarbitone, phenytoin, thiopentone, digoxin, chloroquine and dicoumarol. These studies showed drug protein binding in PEM to be less deranged than might have been expected. Only six drugs, cloxacillin, flucloxacillin, streptomycin, sulphamethoxazole, digoxin and thiopentone, showed a significant decrease in protein binding.

No clinical conclusions could be drawn from these observations for although the free drug concentration may be elevated, the therapeutic effect may not be enhanced since, being free, the drug may be eliminated more rapidly. In addition, diminished renal function in PEM may obviate enhanced elimination [1].

Drug Metabolism

Taking into account the fact that the liver is the main drug metabolising organ and that it is anatomically and functionally deranged in kwashiorkor, it might be expected that drug metabolism would be abnormal in these children. Drug metabolism studies in PEM have fallen into two groups; those looking at therapeutic compounds and those involving marker (non-therapeutic) compounds:

Marker Compound Studies

Hepatic microsomal oxidation has been assessed by studying antipyrine kinetics. The results of Indian [22], Sudanese [17] and South African [10] studies have been similar, showing antipyrine half-life ($t_{1/2}$) to be increased and clearance to be depressed in the acute phase of malnutrition improving with nutritional rehabilitation. Similar observations were made with *D*-glucaric acid excretion, an indirect index of hepatic microsomal activity [18].

D-Glucaric acid excretion increased significantly from 60.6 ± 42.2 to 121.8 ± 105 μmol/24 h over a 3-week nutritional rehabilitation period in 15 children with kwashiorkor [10].

Acetanilide, a further marker substance which is oxidised, was studied in 5 children with kwashiorkor [11]. Results at the time of admission showed a mean $t_{1/2}$ of 4.8 ± 1.07 h and clearance of 0.92 ± 0.19 h^{-1}. After nutritional rehabilitation, $t_{1/2}$ was 1.8 ± 0.22 h^{-1}.

These data imply that hepatic microsomal oxidation/hydroxylation and glucuronidation are depressed in the acute phase of PEM and recover over a 10- to 21-day period of nutritional rehabilitation. They do not, however, provide data on pathways other than oxidation and glucuronidation.

In 1979, *Danhof* et al. [15] showed that different oxidative enzymes (different types of cytochrome P-450) may be involved in the formation of the four primary metabolites of antipyrine, 4-hydroxyantipyrine, norantipyrine, 3-hydroxymethylantipyrine and 3-carboxyantipyrine. This technique

Table III. Mean relative amounts ± SD (% dose) of antipyrine and metabolites in the 24-hour urine samples

	% of dose recovered on admission	% of dose recovered once rehabilitated	p value
Antipyrine	5.2 ± 3.7	2.7 ± 0.9	<0.1
4-Hydroxyantipyrine	6.2 ± 4.5	14.7 ± 5.9	<0.025
Norantipyrine	8.8 ± 5.7	14.3 ± 5.4	>0.1
3-Hydroxymethyl antipyrine	11.8 ± 8.3	20.5 ± 5.6	<0.025
3-Carboxyantipyrine	0.5 ± 0.3	2.0 ± 0.5	<0.0025
Total	32.4 ± 21.9	54.3 ± 8.7	>0.025

was applied to 5 children with kwashiorkor on admission to hospital and on recovery [13]. Results showed a statistically insignificant decrease in antipyrine $t_{1/2}$ from 9.9 ± 3.3 h on admission to 6.8 ± 1.1 h on recovery. This was associated with a significant increase in antipyrine clearance from 0.62 ± 0.13 to 1.07 ± 0.2 ml min^{-1} kg^{-1}. Urinary metabolite results are shown in table III, where it can be seen that for all four metabolites there was an increased output associated with nutritional rehabilitation. This data suggests that the three oxidative pathways of antipyrine seem to be equally affected in children with kwashiorkor. The extrapolation of data from marker compounds, such as antipyrine, to therapeutic compounds, is of limited value as a number of studies have shown poor correlations [27, 28].

Therapeutic Compounds

An early observation that drug metabolism might be affected in kwashiorkor was that of *Wharton and McChesney* [29] who noted that chloroquine was less metabolised in such children than in controls.

Subsequently, *Mehta* et al. [20] have shown chloramphenicol $t_{1/2}$ to be prolonged, clearance diminished and glucuronidation depressed in acute PEM. Hepatic glucuronyl transferase was estimated in some of the children using bilirubin as a substrate and was found to be 30–50% of normal values.

Acetylation has been studied with sulphadiazine in adults and isoniazid in children. With regard to sulphadiazine, *Shastri and Krishnaswamy* [26] studied 6 malnourished adults and 6 controls. They observed sulphadiazine $t_{1/2}$ to be shorter (11.9 ± 1.0 h) in malnourished subjects as opposed to the controls (18.3 ± 1.8 h); this was associated with a 40% increase in the metabolic clearance rate. These results are in contrast to those with isoniazid in 7 patients with kwashiorkor [7] where $t_{1/2}$ was 61.8 ± 20 min and clearance 125.7 ± 7 ml/min on admission changing to 43.8 ± 19.8 min and 329.4 ± 399.6 ml/min on recovery. The observations with isoniazid are of some importance, as this drug is not protein-bound, and thus hypoalbuminaemia and enhanced free drug concentrations cannot have played a part in the altered elimination data.

Oxidation has been studied using phenylbutazone [19]. The results showed undernourished adults to have shorter $t_{1/2}$ (35.9 ± 3.3 h) than did normal smoking adults (48.3 ± 4.2 h) and normal non-smoking adults (56.4 ± 7.6 h). Interpretation of these data is rendered more complex because hepatic and renal function tests were not performed on the subjects. In addition, most of the subjects were agricultural workers and liver function could have been partly induced by insecticide exposure.

There does, however, appear to be a significant difference between results obtained in adults and children. In general, when talking of hepatic drug metabolism in PEM, malnourished adults exhibit enhanced drug clearance, whilst in children it is invariably decreased. There may be three contributing reasons for this: (a) Definitions of malnutrition are not universally accepted and kwashiorkor well nigh never occurs in adults. It is in kwashiorkor that liver function is most severely deranged. (b) Adults are exposed to environmental inducers; smoking, alcohol, insecticides and a wider range of dietary variables [18]. (c) In most paediatric studies, the patients have acted as their own controls. This has not been the case in adults.

Drug Excretion

Once more there is a dichotomy between adult and paediatric data. *Shastri and Krishnaswamy* [25] in a study of 9 well-nourished and 10 undernourished adults showed that when tetracycline was given intravenously $t_{1/2}$ was 7.24 ± 0.6 h in the well-nourished group and 4.1 ± 0.28 h in the undernourished group. This fall in $t_{1/2}$ was associated with a concomitant increase in elimination rate. Whilst the authors have suggested that these results are related to alterations in plasma protein binding, they are difficult to assess as no renal function tests were performed.

Our group studied four antimicrobials, all of which were insignificantly bound to plasma protein and were renally excreted; penicillin [9], gentamicin [8], tobramycin [5] and cefoxitin [12]. In each study, modified para-amino hippuric acid (PAH) clearances, without bladder catheterisation,

Table IV. Pharmacokinetic data for 4 antibiotics and PAH on admission to hospital and after nutritional rehabilitation in children with kwashiorkor

	Half-life, min		Clearance, ml/min	
	admission	recovery	admission	recovery
Penicillin	57.2 ± 20.6	31.6 ± 7.4	183.4 ± 123.3	286.3 ± 80.7
Tobramycin	67.3 ± 18.9	50.2 ± 9.3	–	–
Gentamicin	229 ± 94.8	178.5 ± 99.5	13.6 ± 6.0	28.7 ± 21.3
Cefoxitin	29.2 ± 3.6	28.4 ± 4.6	50.7 ± 5.0	70.6 ± 16.6
PAH	64.3 ± 11.5	48.9 ± 14.7	81.5 ± 22.7	182.3 ± 95.1

were performed as a rough assessment of renal function since it is known that children with PEM have diminished renal plasma flow and glomerular filtration rate [1]. The results of all these studies are similar and are depicted in composite form in table IV. It can be seen that with the exception of cefoxitin, $t_{1/2}$ was significantly prolonged at the time of admission to hospital compared to recovery. With all the drugs, clearance increased with recovery.

In children, it would appear that the pathophysiological alterations known to occur with kwashiorkor are reflected by retention of renally excreted drugs. These changes revert to normal after approximately 10 days of nutritional rehabilitation and certainly by 21 days [3]. With none of the drugs studied was there evidence of toxic serum concentrations being achieved, although multiple dose studies were not carried out.

Conclusions

The present review has referred only to human data. It has been demonstrated that there are a number of pharmacokinetic aberrations in PEM which are related to hepatic and renal dysfunction and changes in plasma protein binding. However, it has not been demonstrated conclusively that these aberrations are of clinical significance.

The basic premise that the cause of mortality in these children may have been 'inappropriate therapy' has not been proven. There are at present no good indications to modify drug dosages in PEM from those given to well-nourished children, except perhaps in instances of therapeutic failure when serum drug level monitoring should be performed, as would be the case in any other patient.

References

1 Alleyne, G.A.O.: The effect of severe protein calorie malnutrition on the renal function of Jamaican children. Pediatrics, Springfield *39:* 400–411 (1967).
2 Bengoa, J.M.: The problem of malnutrition. WHO Chron. *28:* 3–7 (1974).
3 Buchanan, N.; Hansen, J.D.L.; Van der Walt, L.A.; Robinson, R.; Koornhof, H.J.: Chloramphenicol metabolism in children with P.C.M. Am. J. clin. Nutr. *29:* 327–328 (1976).
4 Buchanan, N.: Drug protein binding and protein energy malnutrition. S. Afr. med. J. *52:* 633–737 (1977).

5 Buchanan, N.; Eyberg, C.: Intramuscular tobramycin administration in kwashiorkor. S. Afr. med. J. *53:* 273–274 (1978).
6 Buchanan, N.: Drug kinetics in protein energy malnutrition. S. Afr. med. J. *53:* 327–330 (1978).
7 Buchanan, N.; Eyberg, C.; Davis, M.D.: Isoniazid pharmacokinetics in kwashiorkor. S. Afr. med. J. *56:* 299–300 (1979).
8 Buchanan, N.; Davis, M.D.; Eyberg, C.: Gentamicin pharmacokinetics in kwashiorkor. Br. J. clin. Pharmacol. *8:* 451–453 (1979).
9 Buchanan, N.; Robinson, R.; Koornhof, H.J.; Eyberg, C.: Penicillin pharmacokinetics in kwashiorkor. Am. J. clin. Nutr. *32:* 2233–2236 (1979).
10 Buchanan, N.; Eyberg, C.; Davis, M.D.: Antipyrine pharmacokinetics and *D*-glucaric acid excretion in kwashiorkor. Am. J. clin. Nutr. *32:* 2439–2442 (1979).
11 Buchanan, N.; Davis, M.D.; Henderson, D.B.; Mucklow, J.C.; Rawlins, M.D.: Acetanilide pharmacokinetics in kwashiorkor. Br. J. clin. Pharmacol. *9:* 525–526 (1980).
12 Buchanan, N.; Mithal, Y.; Witcomb, M.: Cefoxitin: intravenous pharmacokinetics and intramuscular bioavailability in kwashiorkor. Br. J. clin. Pharmacol. *9:* 623–627 (1980).
13 Buchanan, N.; Davis, M.; Danhof, M.; Breimer, D.D.: Antipyrine metabolite formation in children in the acute phase of malnutrition and after recovery. Br. J. clin. Pharmacol. *10:* 363–368 (1980).
14 Conney, A.H.; Pantuck, E.J.; Kuntzman, R.; Kappas, A.; Anderson, K.E.; Alvares, A.P.: Nutrition and chemical biotransformations in man. Clin. Pharmacol. Ther. *22:* 707–719 (1977).
15 Danhof, M.; Krom, D.P.; Breimer, D.D.: Studies on the different metabolic pathways of antipyrine in rats: the influence of phenobarbital and 3-methylcholanthrine treatment. Xenobiotica *9:* 695–702 (1979).
16 FAO/WHO: Expert Committee on Nutrition – Eighth report. WHO technical report series, No. 477 (WHO, Geneva 1971).
17 Homeida, M.; Karrar, Z.A.; Roberts, C.J.C.: Drug metabolism in malnourished children. A study with antipyrine. Archs Dis. Childh. *54:* 299–302 (1979).
18 Hunter, J.; Maxwell, J.D.; Corella, M.; Stewart, D.A.; Williams, R.: Urinary *D*-glucaric acid as a test for hepatic enzyme induction in man. Lancet *i:* 572–575 (1971).
19 Krishnaswamy, K.; Ushasri, V.; Niadu, A.N.: The effect of malnutrition on the pharmacokinetics of phenylbutazone. Clin. Pharmacokinet. *6:* 152–159 (1981).
20 Mehta, S.; Kalsi, H.K.; Jayaraman, S.; Mathur, V.S.: Chloramphenicol metabolism in children with protein-calorie malnutrition. Am. J. clin. Nutr. *28:* 977–981 (1975).
21 Mönckeberg, F.; Bravo, M.; Gonzales, O.: Drug metabolism and infantile undernutrition. Nutrition and drug interrelations (Academic Press, New York 1978).
22 Narang, R.K.; Mehta, S.; Mathur, V.S.: Pharmacokinetic study of antipyrine in malnourished children. Am. J. clin. Nutr. *30:* 1979–1982 (1977).
23 Potgieter, J.M.; Hones, M.; Kench, J.E.: The aminoacid composition of serum albumin in patients suffering from kwashiorkor. Clinica chim. Acta *18:* 107–116 (1967).

24 Raghuram, T.C.; Krishnaswamy, K.: Tetracycline absorption in malnutrition. Drug-Nutr. Interact. *1:* 23–29 (1981).
25 Shastri, A.K.; Krishnaswamy, K.: Undernutrition and tetracycline half life. Clinica chim. Acta *66:* 157–164 (1976).
26 Shastri, R.A.; Krishnaswamy, K.: Metabolism of sulphadiazine in malnutrition. Br. J. clin. Pharmacol. *7:* 69–73 (1979).
27 Sjöqvist, F.; Bahr, C. von: Inter-individual differences in drug oxidation: clinical importance. Drug Metab. Disposit. *1:* 469–482 (1973).
28 Vessell, E.S.; Page, J.G.: Genetic control of dicomarol levels in man. J. clin. Invest. *47:* 2657–2663 (1968).
29 Wharton, B.A.; McChesney, E.W.: Chloroquine metabolism in kwashiorkor. J. trop. Pediat. *16:* 130–132 (1970).

N. Buchanan, PhD, FRACP, Department of Paediatrics, University of Sydney
Westmead Centre, Westmead, Sydney N.S.W. 2145 (Australia)

Wld Rev. Nutr. Diet., vol. 43, pp. 140–152 (Karger, Basel 1984)

Interactions between Nutrition, Food and Drugs in Man

R. Roncucci, M. Verry, J.P. Jeanniot
SANOFI-Recherche, Paris, France

Introduction

Metabolic and pharmacokinetic studies in the pharmaceutical industry are aimed at investigating the absorption, distribution, metabolism and elimination (ADME) of drugs. These studies have had three main stages of development. The first stage, which finished during the 1960s, had an essentially promotional aim and its practical medical significance was limited. This first stage was nevertheless the seed of the second stage of development – the stage with which we are still involved – which was aimed to understand and explain the drug's fate in the body and, thus, leading to better orientation of the use of drugs.

The knowledge acquired during these ADME studies in the field of medicinal chemistry make it possible now to envisage the development of the third phase, the so-called 'active' stage, during which new molecules will be conceived and synthesized, taking into account their potential biotransformation and kinetics. This new phase should permit a more rational use of drugs, helping the choice of dosage in order to achieve a higher therapeutic efficiency. The ADME studies have evolved very rapidly and positively as concerns their methods and techniques. However, investigation of the various factors affecting the activity of drugs has not undergone a similar advance. There definitely exist many interactions between a drug and physiological or physiopathological, dietary and environmental factors and factors related to nutritional diseases [1] (table I).

Some of these parameters have been studied in depth although detailed studies were often with limited targets. This is the case, for example, with

Table I. Main factors affecting drug disposition [1]

Intrinsic factors	Extrinsic factors
Sex	due to drug
Age	formulation factors route of administration
Genetic factors	time of administration
Various pathological states Liver or renal insufficiency, cardiovascular diseases, fever, hormonal state, malnutrition	drug interactions
	independent of drug food smoking
Pregnancy	drinks food additives
Circadian rhythms	environmental pollutants
Menstrual rhythms	enzyme inhibition or induction climatic conditions noise

ADME studies in renal or hepatic insufficiency or studies researching the influence of new formulations on the bioavailability of drugs.

On the other hand, it must be noted that interactions between nutrition, food and ADME studies of drugs have up to now only produced results with a limited general significance. Furthermore, these gaps contrast with the normal recommendations about when drugs should be taken in relation to mealtime. Within this context the essential merit of this symposium was to demonstrate the interest of undertaking such interaction studies and to shed some light on an area which is still very dark.

Principal Factors Affecting the Metabolic Fate of Drugs

The plenary conferences and the papers presented during the course of this symposium can be brought together in three major groups of factors which can modify a drug's fate in the body (fig. 1).

One important group of these factors is food. Breast milk was included in this group as a nutrient carrier of the drugs taken by the mother. So it is important to assess the potential risk reaching the infant through breast milk. The second category of factors considered concerns the *environment.* New and important information was presented about the effects of some

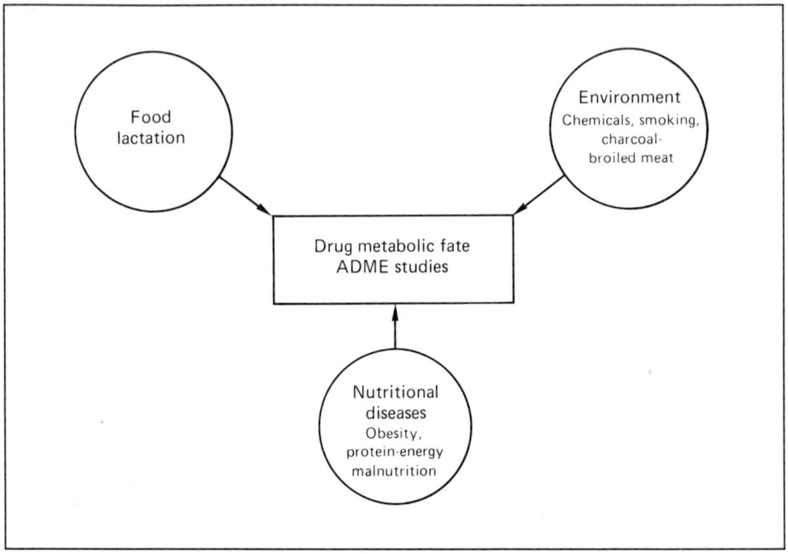

Fig. 1. Major factors affecting the metabolic fate of drugs.

environmental chemical pollutants, such as heavy metals and certain insecticides. Smoking, alcohol and the way of cooking food can also have important repercussions on certain pharmacological agents. The third and last group of factors concerns the effects of certain *nutritional diseases* such as obesity and protein-energy malnutrition. This is still a little studied field, which ought to merit more extensive investigation. Among the numerous factors which affect the fate of drugs these parameters are decisive enough to have focussed the theme of this symposium.

Dietary Factors

The effect of food on the rate of absorption and bioavailability of drugs has been the purpose of numerous studies. *Welling* [2, 3] reviewed the observed effects and some examples are cited in table II.

In most cases, the absorption of drugs from the gastrointestinal tract is reduced or delayed by food. However, some drugs are unaffected by food (theophylline, nitrazepam, warfarin) while the absorption of a small number of drugs is increased (griseofulvin, phenytoin, dicoumarol).

Table II. Drugs whose absorption has been reported to be reduced, delayed or increased by food [3]

Reduced	Delayed	Increased
Many	many	some
Erythromycins	cephalosporins	erythromycins
Penicillins	erythromycin	griseofulvin
Tetracyclines	many	nitrofurantoin
Rifampicine	sulfamides	diazepam
Antipyrine	furosemide	dicoumarol
Aspirin	acetaminophen	hydralazine
Phenacetin	alclofenac	hydrochlorothiazide
Isoniazid	cimetidine	lithium
Levodopa	digoxin	propranolol
Propantheline	indoprofen	metoprolol
Solatol	potassium	phenytoin
Theophylline		riboflavin
		spironolactone

Some other examples borrowed from the literature clearly illustrate the modifications to the absorption of a drug, depending on whether the drug is taken fasting or during a meal.

The bioavailability of alclofenac, a non-steroidal anti-inflammatory agent, is greatly reduced when administered orally after a meal [4]. Figure 2 shows that the area under the curve of plasma concentrations of an unchanged drug as a function of time is reduced by approximately one third simply when taken with food.

Welling [3] showed that in the case of aspirin, not only its bioavailability was reduced when taken with food, but also the time to reach the peak plasma level was significantly delayed, especially after a high carbohydrate meal (fig. 3). The results shown by *Melander* [this volume] confirm these observations. However, he notes that it is currently impossible to predict, on a theoretical basis, the influence of food intake on the bioavailability of drugs. Results presented on β-blockers underline the disparity of these interactions, even within a relatively homogeneous chemical family.

Melander [this volume], as well as *Welling* [2, 3], suggests that food intake may influence the absorption of drugs by a possible modification of the presystemic hepatic drug metabolism. For example, concomitant food intake can induce the deacetylation of atenolol during its absorption and thus largely reduce the bioavailability of this drug. In the same conditions,

2

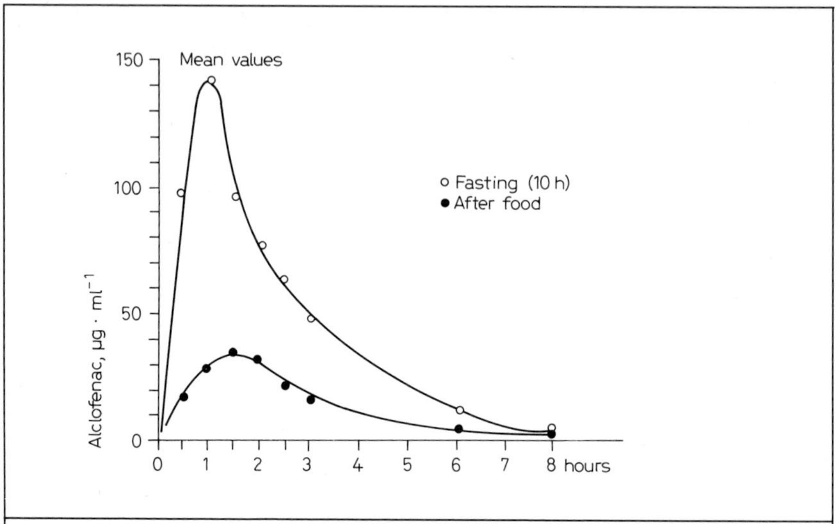

3

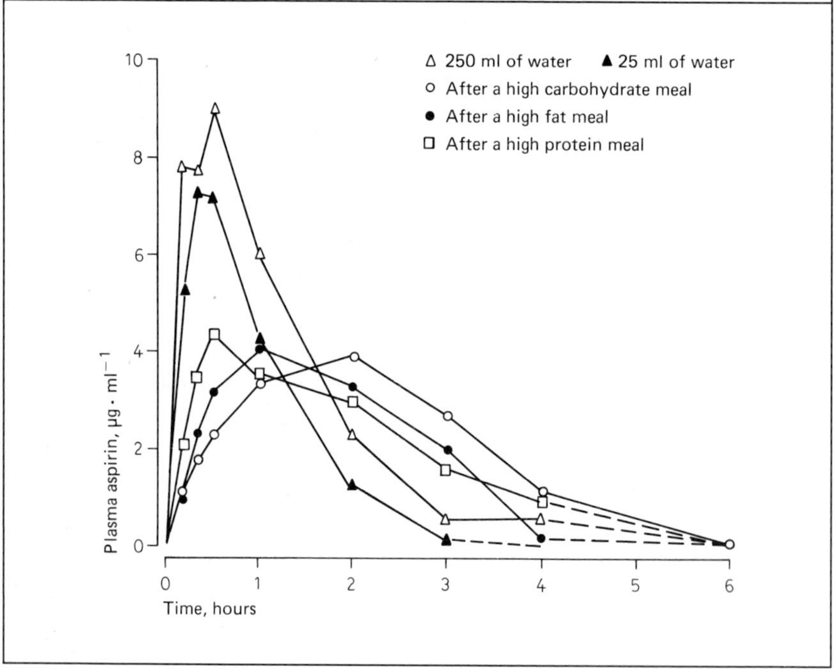

Fig. 2. Effect of food an alclofenac bioavailability [4]. Alclofenac plasma levels in 4 healthy volunteers after oral intake of 1 g of the drug as tablets.

Fig. 3. Influence of nutritional factors on plasma levels of aspirin (single oral dose, 650 mg) [3].

Table III. Interactions between nutrients and drugs in the gastrointestinal tract

Drug binding to food components
Effects of food on
Gastrointestinal transit
Passage across membranes
First pass effect
Biliary flow

the bioavailability of propranolol is increased. In this respect the original studies performed by *Bernier* et al. on the human assay of site and absorption rate of drugs, particularly illustrative for metoprolol, have to be mentioned. However, dietary variations in the bioavailability of drugs have numerous and complex causes. Some of these have been collected in table III.

Food may play a role of drug carrier from gastrointestinal tract to systemic blood, as emphasized by *Roe* [this volume]. Water-soluble substances, which are absorbed by an active transport mechanism, are better absorbed with a concomitant high carbohydrate meal; such is the case of riboflavin (vitamin B_2), a water-soluble vitamin. On the contrary, fat-soluble vitamins (β-carotene, retinal) have their absorption enhanced by fat ingestion as lecithin or α-tocopherol. The biliary flow which is increased by a high fat meal enhances micelle formation and thus fat-soluble compound absorption.

Another important factor is the effect of food on the increased rate of the splanchnic and hepatic blood flow. In fact, fat-soluble drugs remain a short time in contact with the gastrointestinal mucosa and the liver, so these drugs are less metabolized during the first pass through the liver and are more rapidly eliminated from the presystemic area.

Moreover, the nutritional status may also influence the protein-binding characteristics of a drug, as has been demonstrated by *Gayte-Sorbier and Airando* [this volume].

Remembering that only the free fraction of a drug (not bound to proteins) is pharmacologically active, one easily understands the interest of such studies. For example, the binding of valproic acid significantly changes according to the palmitic acid/albumin ratio, present in serum. The binding percentage of several cephalosporins changes with the blood levels of free fatty acids and with the length of the fatty acid chain.

Table IV. Drug excretion in milk

Factors governing drug concentration in breast milk	Characteristics of nursing infants
Dose	volume of distribution different from that observed in adult
Free fraction of drug	immature neonatal liver
Molecular weight	risks due to defects in biotransformation and excretion
Fat solubility	
Ionization	
pH gradient between plasma and milk	

We must also keep in mind the possibility of drug binding with food itself, for example interactions between milk and cheese and certain antibiotics (several tetracyclins, penicillins and erythromycin): the calcium ions contained in these dairy products form nonabsorbed complexes with these drugs [5].

Kirskey and Groziak [this volume] underlined the potential risks of using drugs during lactation. Table IV shows factors conditioning excretion of drugs in breast milk. According to these authors, it is only the free fraction of a drug which is excreted in breast milk. Recently, basic concepts regarding milk formation, accumulation of drugs in breast milk and the extent of exposure of the infant to the drugs ingested by the mother have been reviewed [6]. This problem is particularly acute for the newborn child, not only because of the immaturity of its detoxification and excretion systems, but also because of the differences in the binding rate to proteins and the volumes of distribution.

Environmental Factors

In this second class of factors, the following will be considered: alcohol, tea, coffee, smoking, oral contraceptives, environmental pollutants and the effect of a charcoal-broiled diet on the pharmacokinetic parameters of drugs. These interactions were little mentioned during this symposium but nevertheless deserve our attention.

Let us first consider the interactions between drugs and acute or chronic *alcohol* ingestion. These interactions have been involved in several studies which were recently reviewed in the literature [7, 8].

Acute and chronic alcohol ingestion can alter both the pharmacodynamics and pharmacokinetics of drugs. Modification on drug alcohol is the most important for psychotherapeutic drugs and drugs having side effects on the central nervous system.

The excitatory followed by the depressive effect of alcohol affects sensory and intellectual functions then vigilance and autonomic functions. There may, therefore, exist interactions with numerous drugs.

Generally, sedatives have their action enhance by alcohol (tranquillizers, neuroleptics, some antidepressants). In the same way, hypnotic, analgesic, antihistamine or anticonvulsant agents may be potentiated to the extent of causing coma when alcohol is taken simultaneously.

Chronic alcohol ingestion also induces drug metabolism, causing smooth endoplasmic reticulum proliferation and greatly increasing hepatic microsomal activities and cytochrome P-450. The clinical consequences of such interactions are extremely variable. They depend on the amount of alcohol ingested, the kinetics of ethanol being dose-dependent, the metabolic and pharmacokinetic characteristics of the drug (hepatic extraction ratio, protein binding, and volume of distribution).

Until now, few systematic studies of the mechanism of alcohol-drug interaction have been reported. Such studies should be considered, measuring the parent drug and its metabolites in the body and correlating them with the pharmacological action in such a way as to determine the clinical significance of observed metabolic and kinetic changes.

The interaction between drugs and *tea* or *coffee* retains an increasing attention [9, 10]. Some results obtained with phenothiazines show that a substantial proportion of orally administered drug may be precipitated as a highly insoluble compound if coffee or, more especially, tea is taken close to drug administration. Interactions between caffein and barbiturates have been reported [10]. Particular attention should be paid to the effect of an excessive coffee consumption accompanying oral ingestion of neuroleptics, anxiolytics, hypnotics, antidepressants or monoamine oxidase (MAO) inhibiting agents.

On the other hand, interactions may exist between *oral contraceptives* and drugs. These interactions are suspected but are yet little known. Thus, induction of hepatic microsomes by some drugs may alter or increase the rate of biotransformation of steroid contraceptives and affect their action. Inducing drugs, such as barbiturates or rifampicin, were thought to provoke metrorrhagia in women treated by oral contraceptives. A significant decrease of nitrazepam clearance and more especially intrinsic clearance of the

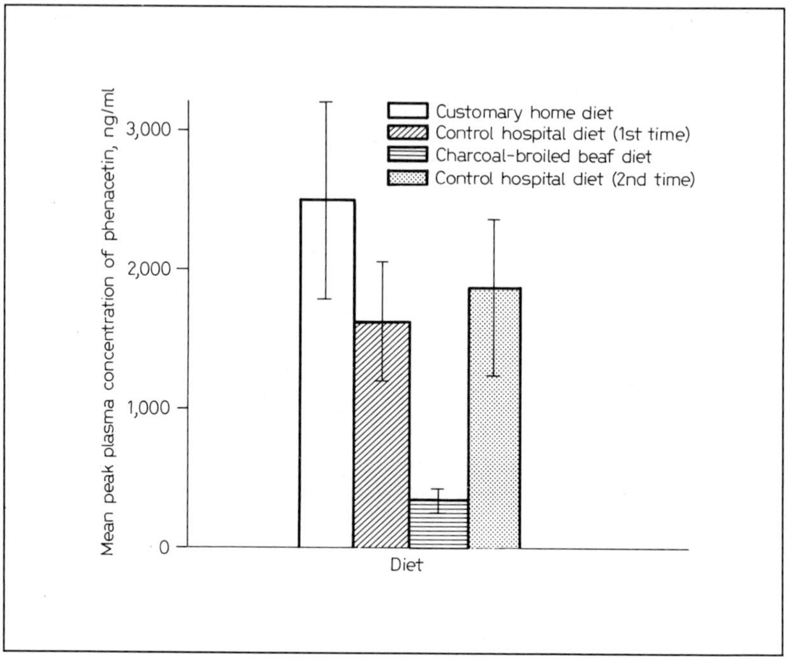

Fig. 4. Effect of a charcoal-broiled beef diet on the peak plasma concentration of phenacetin in humans. Phenacetin (900 mg) was administered orally to 9 subjects after each dietary regimen [12].

free fraction of the drug was observed in young women using oral contraceptives [11].

Alvares [this volume] has shown that factors as different as exposure to *heavy metals* (lead, cadmium) or to *insecticides* and *pesticides* (polychlorinated compounds) or to *cigarette* smoking can result in modifications of drug metabolism. These authors explain the wide variety of these interactions by common mechanisms based on induction of microsomal enzymes. A clearly demonstrated example of such interactions was reported concerning the effect of *charcoal-broiled* beef on the metabolism of phenacetin in the rat. These observations were confirmed in man by *Conney* et al. [12]. In volunteers eating a diet containing charcoal-broiled beef for 4 days, a markedly lowered area under the plasma concentration time curves of phenacetin is shown (fig. 4). The results suggest that charcoal-broiled beef, a food which contains high concentrations of polycyclic hydrocarbons, induces the metabolism of phenacetin in the gastrointestinal tract and/or during its first pass through the liver. *Conney* et al. [12] suggest that the amount of polycyclic hydrocarbons ingested with a charcoal-broiled steak is equivalent to 5–10 packets of cigarettes. These studies show that environmental factors can play an important role on the fate of drugs in the body, especially by modifying metabolism by induction of inhibition of enzyme systems involved in biotransformation.

Nutritional Disease and Drug Interactions

In this last group of factors capable of modifying the drug's fate, we will study the influence of obesity and protein caloric malnutrition. *Obesity,* although it does not have major influence on the absorption phenomena, is on the other hand responsible for some important modifications in distribution, metabolism and elimination of drugs. The volume of distribution, the elimination half-life and to a lesser extent the body clearance, are the pharmacokinetic parameters which can be altered in obesity.

The distribution of a drug depends mainly on its lipid solubility. Thus, drugs with high lipid solubility may be expected to be distributed more extensively in subjects with excess body weight than in those with ideal body weight. This relationship between drug distribution and drug lipid solubility was well pointed out, comparing pharmacokinetics of diazepam and antipyrine in obese and normal body weight subjects [13, 14]. The results are illustrated in table V.

The influence of obesity was tested comparing the volume of distribution of antipyrine, a highly water-soluble drug, essentially distributed in aqueous fluids with that of diazepam, a highly lipophilic drug widely distributed in fat. The effect of obesity on the volume of distribution is shown in table V. The influence is particularly marked for diazepam. Its distributional change in obesity is also accompanied by a significant change of the elimination half-life. This latter is considerably increased in obesity.

In the case of some drugs, these results suggest that their dosage must be adjusted in obese subjects. The results reported by *Buchanan* and *Shastri* [this volume] showed the effects of *malnutrition* on drug pharmacokinetics. As previously mentioned by *Krishnaswamy* [15], protein caloric malnutrition is usually complex and many deficiencies occur simultaneously. Changes occur in almost every organ of the body and the main physiological

Table V. Pharmacokinetic parameters of antipyrine and diazepam in obese and normal body weight subjects [14]

	Antipyrine		Diazepam	
	control (n = 25)	obese (n = 23)	control (n = 17)	obese (n = 17)
T ½ β (h)	10.7	15**	40	95*
Volume of distribution, liters	39.7	44.9	90.7	291.9*
Clearance, ml/min	47.6	38	27.3	38.1**

* $p < 0.001$; ** $p < 0.005$.

functions are affected. The functional status of the gastrointestinal tract is markedly altered by gastric dilatation and ptosis, gastric mucosal atrophy, hypochlorhydria and modification of transit time.

Protein-binding of drugs is affected by hypoalbuminemia which occurs in the majority of malnourished individuals. On the other hand, globulin levels are increased during infections while lipoproteins are reduced. Hypoalbuminemia leads to less binding of some drugs and to an increasing free fraction in plasma with a potential risk of over dosage.

The hepatic changes in malnutrition may alter xenobiotic metabolism. The liver shows functional damage and deficiencies in proteins, minerals, and vitamins modify microsomal enzyme activities.

Finally, in malnutrition at least in its severe forms, changes in glomerular filtration, tubular secretion, and abnormalities in biliary excretion may be encountered. So the elimination of drugs can be greatly modified. Thus, in malnutrition and especially in kwashiorkor, the most severe form of caloric malnutrition, numerous physiopathological changes occur which alter drug metabolism and kinetics. Drugs are being widely used to treat infections and illness which coexist with malnutrition. Also, the physician must be aware of drug dosing in malnourished individuals. Therefore, systematic kinetic studies must be undertaken in various nutritional deficiency disorders. Evaluation of drug kinetics and metabolism in malnutrition will enable us to have a more rational therapeutic approach and help to reduce side effects.

Conclusion

We have tried to bring together the principal messages of this symposium in three major themes. However, this review cannot reflect all the papers presented. It is comforting to note that great progress has been made in the knowledge and therefore in the control of food and environmental factors, which can influence the drug's fate. This knowledge should enable the physician to use better dosage schedules and thus enable him to reach better definitions of the risk/benefit ratios of drugs. Nevertheless, the interactions necessarily existing between the various recognized factors have only been studied in a few, rare cases and systematic studies aimed at a wider understanding of the implied mechanisms would be very desirable.

As far as possible, preclinical experimentation should also progress by the focussing on multiparametric models, reproducing the main nutritional variables. Clinically speaking, the study of biological parameters concerned with food should be taken into account to a much greater extent. In fact, as shown by *Berchtold* et al. [this volume], some dietary foods could play a significant role, notably in the prevention of cardiovascular diseases and cancer.

The growing impact of biotechnologies in the agrobiological field should make the task of the nutritionist easier by offering him well-identified and better-standardized nutrients. In view of the fact that we still have a long way to go with the themes of this international symposium, we should like to express the wish of everyone to see this type of experiment repeated.

Finally, on behalf of the speakers and participants, we would like to thank and congratulate *G. Debry* and the Organization Committee on the success of this symposium.

References

1 Dry, J.: Entretiens de Bichat, Pitié-Salpêtrière Thérapeutique, pp. 133–135 (1978).
2 Welling, P.G.: J. Pharmacokinet. Biopharm. *5:* 291–334 (1977).
3 Welling, P.G.: Pharm. Internat. *1:* 14–18 (1980).
4 Roncucci, R.; Lambelin, G.: Drugs exp. clin. Res. *2:* 9–25 (1977).
5 Bartelink, A.: in Cluff, Petrie, Clinical effects of interactions between drugs, pp. 103–116 (Excerpta Medica, Amsterdam 1974).
6 Welch, R.M.; Findlay, J.M.: Drug Metab. Rev. *12:* 261–277 (1981).
7 Sellers, E.M.; Holloway, M.R.: Clin. Pharmacokinet. *3:* 440–452 (1978).
8 Mezey, E.: Pharmacol. Ther. *14:* 411–430 (1981).

9 Cheeseman, H.J.; Neal, M.J.: Br. J. clin. Pharmacol. *12:* 165–169 (1981).
10 Gallant, C.J.; Macaulay, T.; Chandler, R.F.: Can. Pharm. J. *114:* 212–215 (1981).
11 Jochemsen, R.; Van der Graaff, M.; Boeijinga, J.K.; Breimer, D.D.: Br. J. clin. Pharmacol. *13:* 319–324 (1982).
12 Conney, A.H.; Pantuck, E.J.; Kuntzman, R.; Kappas, A.; Anderson, K.E.; Alvares, A.D.: Clin. Pharmacol. Ther. *22:* 707–720 (1976).
13 Abernethy, D.R.; Greenblatt, D.J.; Divoll, M.; Harmatz, J.S.; Shader, R.I.: J. Pharmac. exp. Ther. *217:* 681–685 (1981).
14 Abernethy, D.R.; Greenblatt, D.J.: Clin. Pharmacokinet. *7:* 108–124 (1982).
15 Krishnaswamy, K.: Clin. Pharmacokinet. *3:* 216–240 (1978).

R. Roncucci, PhD, SANOFI-Recherche,
37, avenue Pierre-1er-de-Serbie, F–75008 Paris (France)

Wld Rev. Nutr. Diet., vol. 43, pp. 153–157 (Karger, Basel 1984)

Action of Vitamin D_3-3β-Sulfate during Lactation in the Rat

L. Cancela, N. Le Boulch, L. Miravet
Inserm U-18, Hôpital Lariboisière, Paris, France

Introduction

Mammals can acquire vitamin D in two ways: in food or by photochemistry. In newborns the nutritional source is the most important. Human babies have a vitamin D requirement of about 10 μg (400 IU) a day [1]. But in human milk, the content of free vitamin D is much smaller (about 1 μg) [2].

From cow or human milk whey, a vitamin D sulfate (SO_4 D_3) has been isolated [3, 4]. It can be kept in the mammalian gland and transmitted by milk to suckling pups, who can hydrolyze it [5]. To clarify the role of SO_4 D_3 present in milk, we have compared the effect, in suckling rat pups, of a free vitamin D or SO_4 D_3 treatment of lactating mothers, deprived of vitamin D during pregnancy.

Material and Methods

50 female rats were fed a rachytic diet (0.47% Ca, 0.3% P, 18% protein, diet 11 [-D] INRA La Minière) for 9 weeks beginning at weaning. After 4 weeks -D they received a tiny amount of vitamin D_3 (2 IU/week) for 5 weeks. Then the rats were divided into two groups: the first one was mated with normal males, the second one was not and served as a control group.

On the 19th day of pregnancy, rats were again divided into two groups: one received 650 pmol/day of free vitamin D_3, the other 650 pmol/day of vitamin D_3 sulfoconjugate (in oily solution, administered orally), and this until the 20th day of lactation. The controls were also divided into two groups and treated in the same way. One extra group of 12 rats was taken at weaning and given a commercial diet (1.5% Ca, 0.9% P, 18% proteins, Extra-Labo-M20). They were mated with normal males at the same time as the other group.

The SO_4 D_3 used was synthesized and purified in the laboratory. The mineral contents of bone ash were determined using the right femur from adult rats and the right femur-tibia-fibula from pups.

Calcium and magnesium were evaluated by atomic absorption over Perkin Elmer 303. Phosphorus was evaluated by colorimetric reaction (Biotrol Kit). Vitamin D metabolites were evaluated by radiocompetition after extraction and purification by high pressure lipid chromatography [6].

Results

The results obtained are reported in table I.

Mineral Contents of Bone Ash. We have observed a significant decrease of bone ash in lactating rats when compared to control non-mated rats of the same age, and this in both normal and treated animals. In litters, the bone ash levels were the same whether the mothers were treated by vitamin D_3 or SO_4 D_3.

We have also observed that calcium levels decreased in all lactating mothers, but only mothers treated with SO_4 D_3 showed a significant decrease in phosphorus and magnesium levels. The only difference observed in litters was an increase in magnesium levels (not shown) when mothers received SO_4 D_3.

Serum Levels of Calcium. In partially vitamin D-deprived rats, the calcium levels were higher in pregnant than in non-pregnant animals. Rats treated with vitamin D, lactating or not, had the same levels of calcium; however, when they received SO_4 D_3, the calcium levels were lower in lactating rats. In litters, calcium levels were lower when mothers received SO_4 D_3.

Serum Levels of Phosphorus. In partially vitamin D-deprived rats, phosphorus levels were higher in pregnant than in non-pregnant animals.

Phosphorus levels were no different in lactating or non-lactating animals who received the same treatment. But in adults, as well as in litters, phosphorus levels were significantly lower when they received the SO_4 D_3.

Serum Levels of Vitamin D Metabolites. In partially vitamin D-deprived rats, the 25(OH)D_3 levels were low and no difference was noticed between pregnant and non-pregnant animals. The 1α,25$(OH)_2D_3$ increased in pregnant rats. After vitamin D treatment, the 25(OH)D_3 levels were significantly increased in non-lactating rats but not in lactating animals. The 1α,25$(OH)_2D_3$ was normal in non-lactating rats and increased in lactating rats. After SO_4 D_3 treatment, the 25(OH)D_3 levels were undetectable in both lactating and non-lactating animals; the 1α,25$(OH)_2D_3$ levels were comparable and no significant increase in 1α,25$(OH)_2D_3$ levels was observed in lactating rats. Suckling pups had the same levels of 25(OH)D_3 in both treatments but 1α,25$(OH)_2D_3$ was higher in litters whose mothers received SO_4 D_3.

Table I. Mineral contents (Ca, P) of bone ash, and serum levels of Ca, P and vitamin D metabolites from mother rats, controls and pups

Tr	Mineral contents of bone ash		Serum levels			
	Ca, % BW	P, % BW	Ca, mg/l	P, mg/l	25(OH)D_3 ng/ml	1α,25 $(OH)_2$ D_3 pg/ml
Extra-Labo normal diet						
NP	–	–	103.4±2.1	69.3±3.6	21.4±1.5	83±2.1
P	–	–	112.3±3.4	76.8±3.9	19.5±0.7	119±1
NL	21.2±0.7 } ^{c}	10.6±0.3	105±1.3	62.3±4.1	21.4±1.0	70.8±2.6 } ^{c}
L	15.8±0.4 }	10.3±0.2	103±2.2	57.3±2.4	19.8±0.5	198±2.1 }
Pups	9.3±0.6	6.4±0.12	114.3±0.8	107.8±1.7	13.6±0.7	105.8±9.5
-D diet						
NP	–	–	96.8±1.4 } ^{d}	50.6±1.7 } ^{d}	2.5±0.1	49.1±3.9 } ^{d}
P	–	–	109.8±1.8 }	64±1.8 }	2.0±0.2	107.7±4 }
NL + D_3	18.2±0.5 } ^{a}	10.3±0.3	104.4±1.5	63.2±0.9	9.1±0.6 } ^{d}	60.6±4 } ^{d}
L + D_3	16±0.9 }	10.4±0.3	100.6±1.4	64.6±1.7	1.9±0.08 }	176±13.8 }
NL + SD_3	17.9±0.6 } ^{c}	10.6±0.2 } ^{c}	96.8±0.6 } ^{d}	53±2.6	<1	74.5±13
L + SD_3	14.3±0.5 }	8.5±0.4 }	71.2±3.6 }	52.8±1.8	<1	101±6.2
Pups						
+D_3	9.2±00.4	6.3±0.06	113.9±0.6 } ^{d}	99.5±1.8 } ^{d}	4.7±0.4	102.7±11 } ^{e}
+ SD_3	9.1±0.3	6.1±0.09	108.3±1.1 }	88.7±1.4 }	4.1±0.3	163±14.9 }

NP = Not pregnant; P = pregnant; NL = not lactating; L = lactating; Tr = treatment; BW = bone weight; SD_3 = SO_4 D_3.
Mean ± SEM.
^{a} $p < 0.05$; ^{b} $p < 0.02$; ^{c} $p < 0.01$; ^{d} $p < 0.001$.

Discussion and Conclusion

If we compare the results obtained from rats treated by vitamin D with those from normal rats, receiving the normal Extra-Labo diet, the only difference noticed was the lower levels of vitamin D metabolites in rats treated by vitamin D. This difference is, in fact, due to the higher amounts of vitamin D received by rats fed a normal diet. We have observed that the 650 pmol/day (10 IU) given to rats treated by vitamin D was enough to prevent vitamin D deficiency.

On the other hand, rats receiving SO_4 D_3 showed clear signs of vitamin D deficiency, which were greater when rats were lactating. Thus, one can assume that adult rats do not use SO_4 D_3 or use it very little and that vitamin D requirements are higher during lactation.

Results obtained lead us to believe that SO_4 D_3 given to mothers has been transmitted to pups in the milk, and that the young rat was able to use it, probably after hydrolysis [5]. In litters whose mothers had received vitamin D_3 or SO_4 D_3, the differences observed in serum levels of calcium, phosphorus and $1\alpha,25(OH)_2D_3$ showed that vitamin D_3 or SO_4 D_3 do not give exactly the same results, and several hypotheses can be proposed: (1) SO_4 D_3 is less active than vitamin D_3, (2) in lactating mothers, treated by SO_4 D_3, the levels of calcium and phosphorus in the milk are decreased at the end of lactation, (3) the amount of milk produced by the mammalian gland is decreased, because of the increase in the mother's deficiency in vitamin D. At the beginning of lactation, in vitamin D-depleted animals, the levels of calcium and phosphorus in milk are normal [7], probably because of a higher mobilization of calcium and phosphorus from bone. But we do not know if this is still the case at the end of lactation when deprivation in vitamin D is greater.

References

1 Food and Nutr. Board. Nat. Res. Council: Recommended dietary allowances; 8th ed., p. 54 (National Academy of Sciences, Washington, 1974).

2 Causeret, J.: La valeur vitaminique des laits animaux. Comparaison avec celle du lait de femme. Annls. Nutr. Aliment *25A:* 313–314 (1971).

3 Sahashi, Y.; Suzuki, T.; Higaki, M.; Asano, T.: Metabolic activities of vitamin D in animals. IX. Configuration and isolation of water-soluble vitamin D sulfate in mammalian milks. Vitamins *34:* 467–469 (1966).

4 Le Boulch, N.; Cancela, L.; Miravet, L.: Cholecalciferol sulfate identification in human milk by HPLC. Steroids *39:* 391–398 (1982).
5 Le Boulch, N.; Marnay-Gulat, C.; Laromiguiere, M.; Miravet, L.; Raoul, Y.: Répartition et évolution de la vitamine D_3 sulfoconjuguée chez la rate gestante ou allaitante. C.r. hebd. Séanc. Acad. Sci., Paris *288D:* 409–412 (1966).
6 Shepard, R.; De Luca, H.F.: Determination of vitamin D and its metabolites in plasma. Meth. Enzym. *67:* 393–413 (1980).
7 Toverud, S.; Boass, A.: Hormonal control of calcium metabolism in lactation. Vitams Horm. *37:* 303–347 (1979).

L. Cancela, Inserm U. 18, Hôpital Lariboisière, 6, rue Guy-Patin,
F–75010 Paris (France)

Wld Rev. Nutr. Diet., vol. 43, pp. 158–163 (Karger, Basel 1984)

Absence of Reproducibility of Glycaemic Excursions Induced by Identical Meals in Diabetic Subjects Connected with an Artificial Pancreas

L. Méjean[a], *J. Louis*[a], *R. Mercier*[b], *A. Guillemart*[b], *P. Toussain*[b], *P. Drouin*[a], *G. Debry*[a]

[a]Unité de Recherches de Nutrition et Diététique de l'Inserm U.59 et Département de Nutrition et des Maladies Métaboliques de l'Université de Nancy I, Nancy; [b]Centre de Recherches Sanofi, Montpellier, France

Insulin-dependent diabetic subjects have to regulate the nature, the amount and the frequency of their food intakes and determine the useful doses of insulin so as to avoid phases of hypo- and hyperglycaemia. Much progress has contributed to improve the expectation of life of these patients. However, it has also shown the relevance of the quality of blood glucose control to prevent possible degenerative complications [6]. Ideally treatment in insulin-dependent diabetic subjects would ensure them over a nycthemeron a glycaemic profile as close as possible to that of normal subjects.

The objective of the present work is to determine whether it is possible to show a reproducibility of the daily insulin need in insulin-dependent diabetic subjects undergoing strict control for physical exercise, food intake and glycaemic equilibrium.

Material and Methods

5 insulin-dependent (4 men and 1 woman) subjects gave their informed consent before they underwent an equilibration of their glycaemia by feedback control using an artificial pancreas Biostator® (GCIIS, Laboratoires Miles, Elkhart, USA) for 50 h according to a previously described protocol

[5]: algorithms used were adapted to each subject and maintained under steady-state conditions throughout the experiment [1].

The subjects are allowed to rest throughout the 50 h of recording; meals and snacks are strictly identical (times of food intakes, amount and quality of the food ingested over the 2 days) and correspond to the usual consumption of the subjects. Only the last 48 h of recording are taken into account for statistical analysis. The study compares the results of the glycaemic profiles and the insulin needs obtained in the course of the two successive periods of 24 h ranging from 10 h on day 1 to 10 h on day 2, and from 10 h on day 2 to 10 h on day 3.

The glycaemic profile is quantized by: the mean value of glycaemia measured at 24-hour intervals; the mean value of the index of *Schlichtkrull* et al. [7]; the mean amplitude of glycaemic excursions (MAGE) [8] calculated on the disturbances of amplitude above 1 standard deviation, and the maximum value of glycaemia for each disturbance (irrespective of the amplitude).

The statistical analysis can be divided into two parts: (1) comparison of the individual plots of disturbances in the course of the two nycthemera of the study, (2) comparison of the indices of glycaemic equilibrium by the method of non-parametric tests [2]. The overall insulin needs were calculated by integrating the values recorded every minute and compared for each subject and for each period of the study.

Results

Individual Plots of the Disturbances in the Course of the Nycthemera of the Study

Figure 1 illustrates the position with time and the amplitude (G_{max}) of the disturbances observed for each subject: similar variations were shown between the 2 days; the major disturbances are found during the diurnal period and are induced by food intakes. It is particularly worthwhile pointing out that for each subject the low intensity spontaneous disturbances are observed during the diurnal period at comparable times.

Comparison of the Overall Parameters Characterizing the Glycaemic Equilibrium (table I)

Significant day-to-day variations are observed in mean glycaemic levels. The amplitude of such variations is, however, not constant from one subject to another: if it is very low in subject No. 1, it is much less pro-

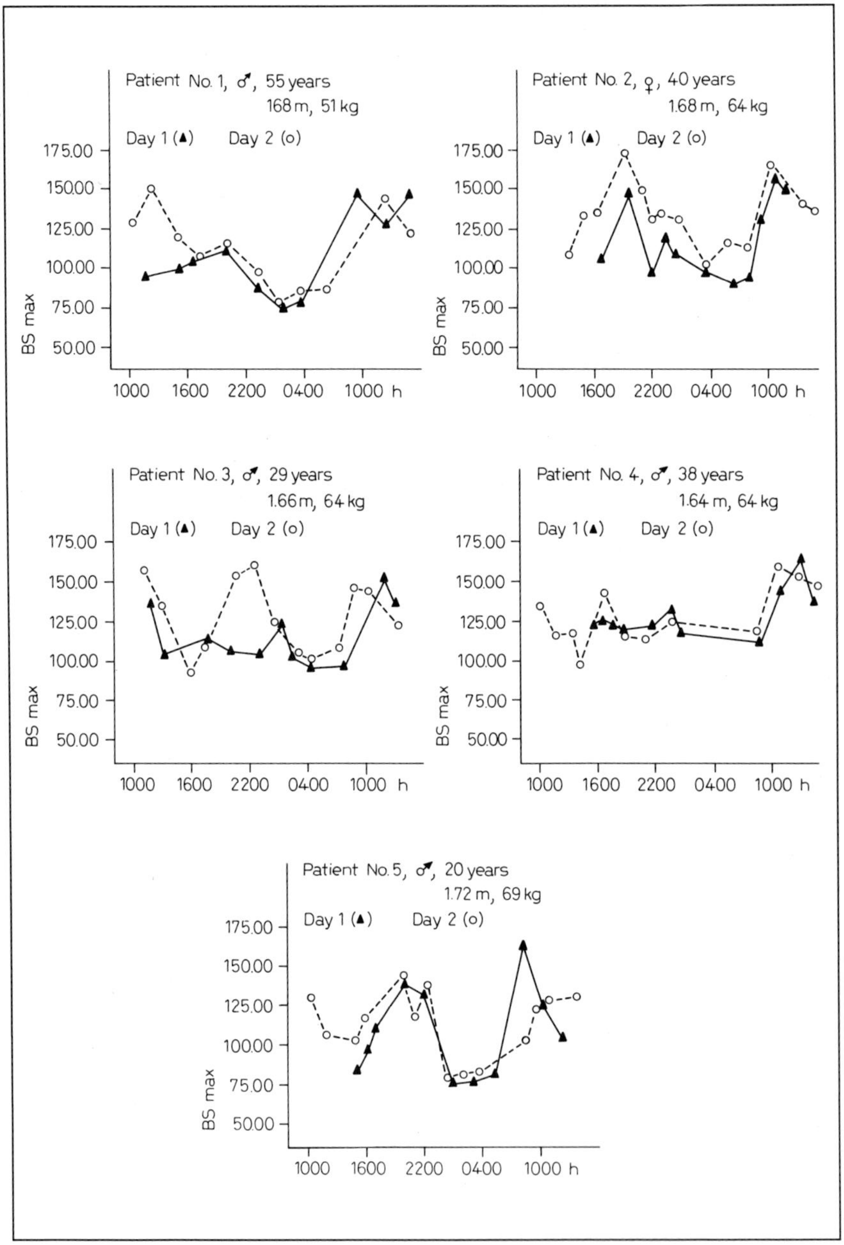

Fig. 1. Profile of disturbances on days 1 and 2. Disturbances are expressed by G_{max} (in mg/dl).

Table I. Comparison of the overall parameters characterizing the glycaemic equilibrium

Subject No.	Mean glycemic levels, mg/dl			Schlichtkrull's index			MAGE index, mg/dl		
	day 1	day 2	signif.	day 1	day 2	signif.	day 1	day 2	signif.
1	94.82	94.66	$p < 0.001$	4.20	2.27	$p < 0.001$	36.0	32.5	–
2	99.33	111.66	$p < 0.001$	3.77	1.48	$p < 0.001$	63.5	41.6	–
3	97.39	105.74	$p < 0.02$	1.97	1.40	$p < 0.001$	39.0	45.4	–
4	115.46	106.54	$p < 0.02$	1.39	1.17	n.s.	78.3	39.3	–
5	89.80	93.80	$p < 0.001$	6.31	2.76	$p < 0.001$	51.8	40.9	–
Mean value	–	–	–	3.53	1.82	–	53.72	39.94	$p < 0.01$

Table II. Overall insulin needs (mean value in mU/day)

Subject No.	Day 1	Day 2
1	60,485	44,752
2	73,074	95,131
3	60,008	95,827
4	100,590	82,413
5	79,555	84,111

nounced in the others. So it is with the direction of these variations which differs from one subject to another. A similar result was obtained with Schlichtkrull's index: the mean value is reduced on day 2. Individual differences are significant in 4 subjects. The mean number of disturbances of amplitude above 1 standard deviation is significantly more marked on day 2 (n = 42) as compared with day 1 (n = 26). The mean amplitude is significantly reduced on day 2.

Comparison of the Overall Insulin Needs

Table II shows individual variations in the overall insulin needs on days 1 and 2. 2 subjects present a reduced need for insulin (subject 1, 26%; subject 4, 18%). The 3 other subjects, however, exhibit an increased need for insulin (subject 2, 30%; subject 3, 60%; subject 5, 6%).

Discussion

The objective of the protocol followed was to assess the reproducibility of insulin needs while maintaining a constancy in the three factors related to the rhythm of life: physical exercise, food intake and the quality of the glycaemic equilibrium.

Three major results emerge from the present work: (1) In spite of the subjection of glycaemic equilibrium to feedback control, spontaneous glycaemic variations are observed, in particular during sleep. These variations are reproducible on a day-to-day basis. This result compares favourably with the existence of circadian variations in blood glucose in glucose tolerance as shown by several authors [3, 4]. (2) The quality of equilibrium is not, however, reproducible in the aggregate or individually: disturbances of low amplitude are of higher occurrence and less pronounced during the second nycthemeron. (3) Although alimentation was strictly controlled and physical activity reduced, the overall need for insulin varies considerably from one day to another and from one subject to another.

The process of automatic control in the treatment of diabetes using the means presently developed (self-checking, programmable injection pump) is still unfit for ensuring to diabetic subjects the levels and nycthemeral variations of glycaemia comparable with those of normal subjects.

References

1 Clemens, A.H.: Artificial beta cell: glucose analyser and control algorithms; in Drouin, Méjean, Debry, Artificial pancreas – clinical applications, pp. 61–77 (Doin, Paris 1979).

2 Dixon, W.J.: BMDP statistical software (University of California Press, Los Angeles 1980).

3 Jarrett, R.J.: Circadian variations in blood glucose levels in glucose tolerance and in plasma immunoreactive insulin levels. Acta diabet. lat. *9:* 263–275 (1972).

4 Owens, D.R.; Wragg, K.G.; Biggs, P.I.; Luzio, S.; Davies, C.J.: The reproducibility of serial meal and oral glucose tolerance tests in normal subjects. Diabète Métab. *7:* 25–33 (1981).

5 Pfeiffer, E.F.: Feedback controlled and preprogrammed insulin infusions in research and treatment of diabetes mellitus. General overview; in Drouin, Méjean, Debry, Artificial pancreas – clinical applications, pp. 13–59 (Doin, Paris 1979).

6 Pirart, J.: Diabète et complications. Présentation d'une étude prospective portant sur 4,000 cas observés entre 1947 et 1973. Diabète Métab. *3:* 173–182 (1977).
7 Schlichtkrull, J.; Funder, J.; Munck, O.: La confrontation des résultats cliniques en diabétologie; in Journées Annuelles de Diabétologie de l'Hôtel Dieu, pp. 143–151 (Flammarion, Paris 1961).
8 Service, F.J.; Molnar, G.D.; Rosevear, J.W.; Ackerman, E.; Gatewood, L.C.; Taylor, W.F.: Mean amplitude of glycemic excursions: a measure of diabetic instability. Diabetes *19:* 644–655 (1970).

L. Méjean, Unité de Recherches de Nutrition et Diététique de l'Inserm U. 59 et Département de Nutrition et des Maladies Métaboliques de l'Université de Nancy I, 40, rue Lionnois, F-54000 Nancy (France)

Wld Rev. Nutr. Diet., vol. 43, pp. 164–169 (Karger, Basel 1984)

Effects of Nonesterified Fatty Acids on the Diethylstilbestrol Binding by Murine and Human Sera and Tissue Proteins

L. Savu, C. Benassayag, G. Vallette, F. Clerc-Hofmann, E.A. Nunez
CNRS ERA 881, Inserm U-224 Faculté X. Bichat, Paris, France

Introduction

Diethylstilbestrol (DES) is a synthetic estrogen analog, widely used in animal studies, and for breeding or clinical purposes. In recent years, administration of this drug to pregnant women has been associated with the development of vaginal adenocarcinoma in the female offspring, but the mechanisms involved in such effects are not elucidated [1].

It is now accepted that the free or protein-bound state of the blood-borne small molecules regulates their biological activities: therefore, it seemed important, for evaluating the physiological impact of DES, to analyze its interactions with the serum proteins of fetus and mother, as well as its relations to metabolites likely to affect the DES-protein interactions, in particular the estradiol-17β (E_2) and the polyunsaturated nonesterified fatty acids (NEFAs) which are able to inhibit the attachment of E_2 to murine α_1-fetoproteins (AFPs) [2] and to the rat estrogen uterine receptor [3]. We summarize below our observations in rat, mouse and man.

Materials and Methods

Sera, Proteins, Uterine Cytosol. Rat and mouse sera were from 19-day pregnant females and fetuses (Sprague-Dawley rats; CD inbred mouse strains; Charles River, France). Human fetuses were 4.5 months old and originated from therapeutic abortions; their sera contained 12% AFP.

Murine AFPs and albumins were purified by preparative gel electrophoresis; human AFP was a gift from Prof. *Nishi* and albumin a Sigma product. The purified proteins were delipidated with charcoal at pH 3 [2]. Rat uterine cytosol was prepared as described [3].

Binding Studies. A gel equilibration technique [4] is applied. We measured: '1/P' binding indices (P is the protein concentration corresponding to bound/free ligand ratios of 1); 'Ka' association constant: 'n' maximum number of binding sites; inhibitory effects of increasing amounts of unlabelled competitors on binding of fixed amounts of [^{3}H] ligand.

Results

'1/P' Binding Indices for DES in Whole Sera and Purified Proteins from Rat, Mouse and Man (table I). The DES binding by whole sera is high in adults and fetuses of the 3 species: however, the human fetus stands out as the weakest binder of the drug.

With the albumin and AFP preparations, DES interacts more strongly than with the sera from which these proteins were purified, but for one exception: the human AFP, which virtually does not bind DES. Thus, AFP and albumin afford major contributions to the association of DES with the rat and mouse fetal sera; on the other hand, albumin alone is responsible for the bulk of the DES-serum interactions in the adults of the three species and in the human fetus.

Table I. Binding indices (1/P, l/g) for DES measured on whole sera and purified serum proteins from different sources [4]

	Rat	Mouse	Human
Fetus	6 ± 4	14 ± 2	3.4 ± 0.5
Normal female	7 ± 3	8 ± 1.5	12 ± 5
Pregnant	6 ± 2	9.5 ± 2	15 ± 3
Serum albumin	24 ± 4	15 ± 1	24 ± 3
α_1-Fetoprotein	31 ± 2	19.5 ± 6	nonmeasurable[1]

[1] By analytical electrophoresis of pure AFP incubated with [^{3}H]DES.

Table II. Equilibrium binding parameters of DES with purified native and delipidated rat AFP and albumin preparations [4]

Binding parameters	Purified AFP preparations		Purified albumin preparations	
	native	delipidated	native	delipidated
Ka × 10^6 M^{-1}	1.3 ± 0.16[1]	1.01 ± 0.1	0.17 ± 0.01[1]	0.12 ± 0.01
N	2.2 ± 0.3[2]	5.6 ± 0.8	11.4 ± 0.5[1]	11 ± 0.3

[1] Difference from delipidated: nonsignificant.
[2] Statistically different from delipidated AFP: $p < 0.001$ by Student's t test.

Binding Parameters of DES with Purified Rat AFP and Albumin. Effects of Delipidation (table II) [4]. Low affinity high capacity characteristics are demonstrated for the interactions of DES with either AFP (Ka ~ 10^6 M^{-1}; n ~ 2) or albumin (Ka ~ 10^5 M^{-1}; n ~ 11).

The removal of the nondialyzable lipids attached to the purified rat AFP increases by a factor of about 3 the number of its apparent DES sites, whereas the delipidation of albumin has little effect on its interaction with DES.

As shown by mass spectrometry/gas chromatography studies from our group [2], the lipid moiety which thus masks part of the DES sites on AFP consists mainly of long chain NEFA. This NEFA fraction also masks an important portion of the high affinity E_2-binding sites of the rat AFP [5].

These results suggest possible interferences of the estrogens and the NEFAs with the binding of DES to murine AFPs. The inhibition studies summarized below will clarify this point.

Inhibition Experiments with Mouse AFP and Albumin [6]. Mutual dose-dependent inhibitions among E_2, DES and the arachidonic acid ($C_{20:4}$), for binding to AFP, are evidenced in figure 1. Bilirubin binding is not influenced by any of these different ligands. By contrast, figure 2 demonstrates that there is no such interference among the four compounds when they interact with albumin. These results suggest a partial overlap (or identity) of the AFP sites involved in the binding of the natural estrogen, its

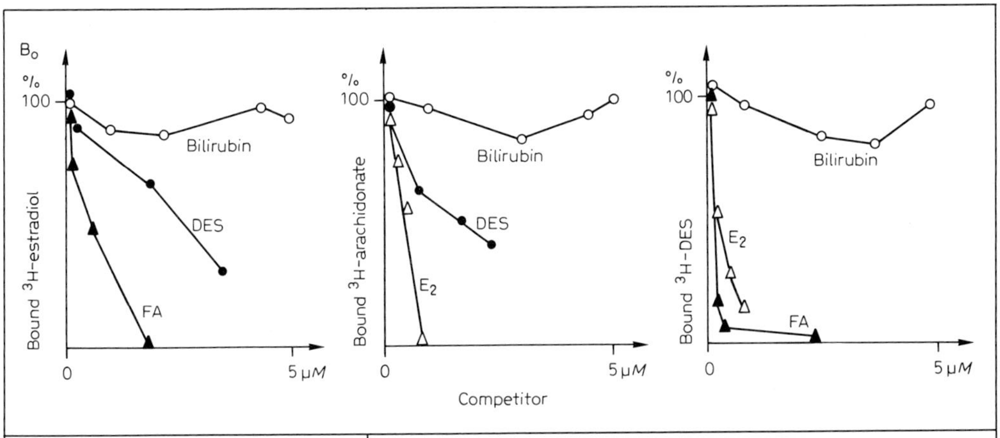

1

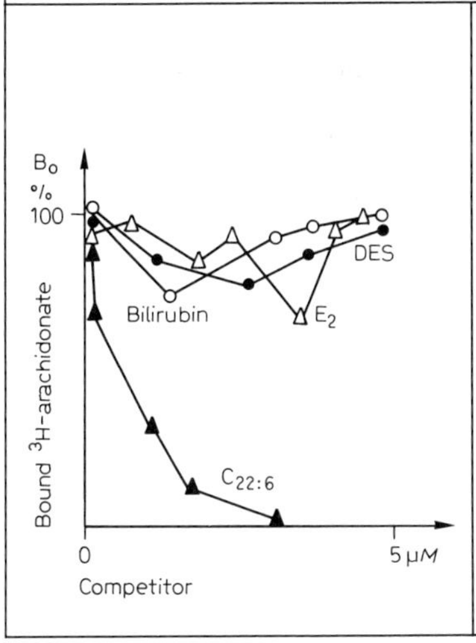

2

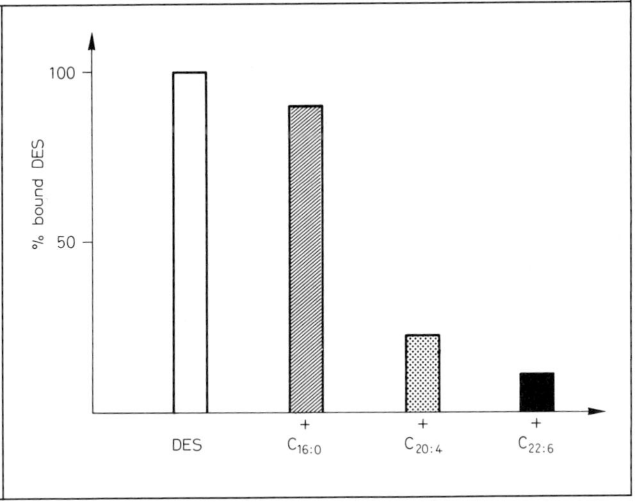

3

Fig. 1. Competition experiments with mouse AFP. Mutual displacements among E_2, DES, NEFA and bilirubin [6].

Fig. 2. Competition experiments with mouse albumin. Effects of DES, E_2, the $C_{22:6}$ fatty acid, and bilirubin on the binding of arachidonate ($C_{20:4}$) to mouse albumin [6].

Fig. 3. Inhibition of the binding of tritiated diethylstilbestrol (^{3}H-DES) to cytosol receptor 8S by saturated and unsaturated NEFA. The binding of ^{3}H-DES ($1 \cdot 10^{-9}$ *M*) to 8S receptor is measured in a 5–20% saccharose gradient after incubation for 2 h at 4 °C of 0.3 ml uterine cytosol from 24-day-old rats (600 μg proteins) with different NEFA: palmitic acid ($C_{16:0}$) ($2.2 \cdot 10^{-4}$ *M*), arachidonic acid ($C_{20:4}$) ($1.9 \cdot 10^{-4}$ *M*), docosahexaenoic acid ($C_{22:6}$) ($1.7 \cdot 10^{-4}$ *M*). The percent of inhibition was calculated after integration of the radioactivity of the bound DES to the peak 8S and subtraction of nonspecific binding. Mean of three determinations.

analog and the fatty acid and designate AFP as a sensitive modulator of the free/bound ratios of its various ligands.

Inhibition Experiments with Rat Uterine Cytosol. NEFA inhibit not only the comparatively weak DES-AFP interaction but also, as shown in figure 3, the strong binding of DES to the estrogen receptors of uterine cytosol. The inhibition appears directly correlated to the unsaturation of the fatty acid, a result consistent with the previously demonstrated NEFA effects on the estrogen-murine AFPs interactions [2] or estrogen-rat uterine receptors [3].

Discussion

A long-lived concept holds that synthetic hormones bind to intracellular hormone receptors but not to plasma proteins. The present studies challenge this notion, by demonstrating elevated interactions of the estrogen analog DES with the serum proteins of rat, mouse and man, whether adult or fetal.

These interactions are age- and species-dependent. Thus, rat and mouse AFPs associate significantly with DES but human AFP does not. This could partly explain the weak protection of estrogen target tissues in human fetus against the circulating DES, and might constitute one of the factors involved in the reported [1] carcinogenic effects of the drug.

A further significant fact revealed by our studies is that the weak murine AFP-DES interaction is able to hamper the strong AFP-E_2 or AFP-NEFA interactions. Therefore, pharmacological amounts of the drug – and, more generally, of any therapeutic compound – may disturb the physiological bound/free equilibria of important endogenous metabolites. The impacts of such disequilibria seem worth investigating whenever pharmacological tests are performed.

Finally, we should like to stress the interest of the mutual inhibitory effects among DES, NEFA and E_2 for binding to uterine receptors, as demonstrated here and previously [3] for the rat. These phenomena suggest important roles for the circulating and tissular lipids in modulating the activities of natural or synthetic estrogen. Thus, it may be envisaged that characteristics of the lipid diet or lipid metabolism in the DES-treated mothers could have aggravated or relieved the undesirable fixation of the drug on fetal targets.

References

1 Ulfelder, H.: The stilboestrol-adenosis-carcinoma syndrome. J. Cancer *38:* 426–431 (1976).

2 Vallette, G.; Benassayag, C.; Savu, L.; Delorme, J.; Nunez, E.A.; Doumas, J.; Maume, G.; Maume, B.F.: The serum competitor of estrogen-rat alpha$_1$-foetoprotein interactions. Identification as a mixture of non-esterified fatty acids. Biochem. J. *187:* 851–856 (1980).

3 Benassayag, G.; Vallette, G.; Savu, L.; Clerc-Hofmann, F.; Christeff, N.; Muller, F.; Delorme, J.; Nunez, E.A.: Relations between serum α_1-foetoprotein and uterine cytosol receptors in the immature rat: importance of fatty acid ligands; in Peeters, Protides of the biological fluids, pp. 369–372 (Pergamon Press, Oxford 1982).

4 Savu, L.; Benassayag, C.; Vallette, G.; Nunez, E.A.: Ligand properties of diethylstilboestrol: studies with purified native and fatty acid-free rat alpha$_1$-foetoprotein and albumin. Steroids *34:* 737–748 (1979).

5 Benassayag, C.; Savu, L.; Vallette, G.; Delorme, J.; Nunez, E.A.: Relations between fatty acids and estrogen binding properties of pure rat alpha$_1$-foetoprotein. Biochim. biophys. Acta *587:* 227–237 (1979).

6 Savu, L.; Benassayag, C.; Vallette, G.; Christeff, N.; Nunez, E.A.: Mouse α_1-fetoprotein and albumin. A comparison of their binding properties with estrogen and fatty acid ligands. J. biol. Chem. *256:* 9414–9418 (1981).

L. Savu, MD, CNRS ERA 881, Inserm U. 224 Faculté X. Bichat, 16, rue Huchard, F–75018 Paris (France)

Wld Rev. Nutr. Diet., vol. 43, pp. 170–173 (Karger, Basel 1984)

Polyunsaturated Fatty Acids: Drug or Food?

F. Driss[a], *P. Darcet*[a], *M. Lagarde*[b], *E. Vericel*[b], *B. Velardo*[b], *M. Guichardent*[b], *M. Dechavanne*[b]

[a]Centre de Gérontologie, Paris; [b]Inserm U-63, Laboratoire d'Hémobiologie, Faculté de Médecine Alexis-Carrel, Lyon, France

Several works have mentioned the relationship between platelet functions, fats and thrombosis. These risk factors could be considered as responsible of the high incidence in coronary and cerebrovascular diseases. The progress slowly realized in the comprehension of these mechanisms stimulates a search for new therapeutic strategies. An alternate strategy, which may have considerable potential, would imply dietary supplementation with polyunsaturated fatty acids. These fatty acids could alter platelet functions and reduce aggregation and thrombotic events.

$C_{20:3\omega6}$, the precursor of PGE_1, was given to young volunteers by *Willis* et al. [1]. The intake of $C_{20:3\omega6}$ increases PGE_1 production and inhibits platelet aggregation [2]. In Greenland Eskimos, it has been reported that the low frequency for cardiovascular disease could be due to their exclusive marine food consumption, which provides high amounts of $C_{20:5\omega3}$ (EPA) and $C_{22:6\omega3}$ [3]. Since this epidemiological study, there were several reports that fish oils containing $C_{20:5\omega3}$ could inhibit platelet aggregation and prolong bleeding [4, 5]. However, feeding studies with $C_{20:5\omega3}$-rich fish oils, in both animals and human volunteers, did not indicate clearly the available doses and periods of the feeding. Furthermore, the question arose whether diets cause undesirable increases in leukotriene/prostaglandin ratio and other secondary effects. We report in the present study, for the first time, results of weak intakes of pure $C_{20:5\omega3}$ in two prethrombotic stages: diabetes mellitus and elderly people.

Eicosapentaenoic Acid Intake in Elderly People

Previous studies have shown that platelets from elderly people present an enhancement of platelet aggregation, sometimes associated with stroke and transient attack [6]. We investigate the effect of EPA intake upon the aggregation and the arachidonate metabolism under thrombin stimulation in platelets. 11 elderly subjects were instructed to take 150 mg/daily of $C_{20:5\omega3}$ for 4 weeks. Subjects took no medication and did no change their cooking habits for 2 weeks and throughout experimental period. Results are shown in table I. After $C_{20:5\omega3}$ intake: platelet agregation induced by either collagen, epinephrine, or low concentrations of adenosine 5′-diphosphate (ADP), was significantly reduced; the main oxygenated products from endogenous arachidonate were decreased, TXB2 formation was 3-fold decreased; the fatty acid composition of total lipids or phospholipids from plasma and platelets was not modified.

Eicosapentaenoic Acid Intake in Diabetes mellitus

Lagarde et al. [7] reported that diabetes mellitus patients present an enhancement of platelet aggregation both in PRP and isolated platelet. Furthermore, in these patients inhibition of platelet aggregation by anti-aggregatory prostaglandins PGE_1, PGD_1 PGI_2 is lower than in controls [8].

In this experiment every diabetic patient ingested 50 mg daily of $C_{20:5\omega3}$ during 2 months. Results are shown in table II. After $C_{20:5\omega3}$ intake: platelet aggregation induced by collagen was significantly reduced; PGE_1 was more efficient to inhibit platelet aggregation (table III); TXB2 formation was half decreased; no modification in the fatty acid composition of both plasma and platelet lipids could be observed.

These findings are different from those obtained by using more than 10-fold amounts of $C_{20:5\omega3}$ intake in young healthy volunteers [4, 5, 9]. Indeed, such large amounts of $C_{20:5\omega3}$ partially displace arachidonic acid from platelet phospholipids. Our study shows that the intake of very low amounts of $C_{20:5\omega3}$ has a potent inhibitory effect on platelet aggregation and thromboxane formation. This effect is obtained without any change in polyunsaturated fatty acid pattern, avoiding peroxide derivative formations. This suggests that $C_{20:5\omega3}$ intake inhibits the arachidonate liberation from platelet phospholipids. However, the mechanism by which such amounts of $C_{20:5\omega3}$ decreases the arachidonic acid liberation remains to be explained.

Table I. Effect of 150 mg $C_{20:5\omega3}$ intake upon platelet aggregation and TXB2 formation in elderly people

	Platelet aggregation induced by collagen: area under curve, cm^2/min (n = 11)	TXB2 formation (gas-liquid chromatography) $\mu g/10^9$ platelets (n = 8)
Before $C_{20:5\omega3}$	33.5 ± 2.7	1.63 ± 1.25
After $C_{20:5\omega3}$	28.6 ± 3.7	0.51 ± 0.68
Paired test	4.8 ± 4.7 $p < 0.01$	1.12 ± 1.29 $p < 0.05$

Table II. Effects of 50 mg $C_{20:5\omega3}$ intake upon platelet aggregation and TXB2 formation in diabetes mellitus patients

	Platelet aggregation induced by collagen	TXB2 nmol/10^9 platelets
Before $C_{20:5\omega3}$	0.40 μg/ml	0.25 ± 0.11
After $C_{20:5\omega3}$	0.61 μg/ml	0.10 ± 0.08
Paired test	0.20 ± 0.05 $p < 0.01$	$p < 0.1$

Table III. Anti-aggregatory effect of PGE_1 upon platelet aggregation induced by collagen before and after $C_{20:5\omega3}$ intake in diabetes mellitus patients (n = 5)

PGE_1 ng/ml	PRP	Platelets
Before $C_{20:5\omega3}$	3.20	1.60
After $C_{20:5\omega3}$	1.70	0.81
Paired test	1.50 ± 0.70 $p < 0.01$	0.79 ± 0.30 $p < 0.01$

Previous studies suggested that the evidence of polyunsaturated fatty acid deficiency in elderly people follows a decrease of Δ6 and Δ5 desaturation activities (the key enzymes involved in the biosynthesis of prostaglandin precursors form essential fatty acids) we have recently reported that this deficiency is correlated with an enhanced platelet aggregation [10]. Thus, the hypothesis may arise that the weak amounts of $C_{20:5\omega3}$ that we have given could just counteract the deficiency.

References

1 Willis, A.L.; Comai, K.; Kuhn, D.L.; Paulsrud, J.: Dihomo-γ-linolenate suppresses platelet aggregation when administered in vitro or in vivo. Prostaglandins *8:* 509 (1974).

2 Kernoff, P.B.A.; Willis, A.L.; Stone, K.J.; Davies, J.A.; McNicol, G.P.: Antithrombotic potential of dihomo-γ-linolenic acid in man. Br. med. J. *ii:* 1441 (1977).

3 Dyerberg, J.; Bang, H.O.; Stoffersen, E.; Moncada, S.; Vane, J.R.: Eicosapentaenoic acid and prevention of thrombosis and atherosclerosis. Lancet *i:* 117–119 (1978).

4 Siess, W.; Scherer, B.; Ahling, B.; Roth, P.; Kurzmann, I.; Weber, P.C.: Platelet membrane fatty acids, platelet aggregation and thromboxane formation during a mackerel diet. Lancet *i:* 441–444 (1980).

5 Thorngren, M.; Gustafson, A.: Effects on 11 weeks increase in dietary eicosapentaenoic acid on bleeding time, lipids and platelet aggregation. Lancet *ii:* 1190–1193 (1981).

6 Sie, P.; Montagut, J.; Blanc, M.; Boneu, B.; Caranobe, C.; Cazard, J.C.; Bierme, R.: Evaluation of some platelet parameters in a group of elderly people. Thromb. Haemostasis *45:* 197–199 (1981).

7 Lagarde, M.; Burtin, M.; Berciaud, P.; Blanc, M.; Velardo, B.; Dechavanne, M.: Increase of platelet TXA2 formation and its plasmatic half-life in diabetes mellitus. Thromb. Res. *19:* 823–830 (1980).

8 Lagarde, M.; Berciaud, P.; Burtin, M.; Dechavanne, M.: Refractoriness of diabetic platelet to inhibitory prostaglandins. Prostaglandins Med. *7:* 341–347 (1981).

9 Brox, J.H.; Killie, J.E.; Gunnes, S.; Nordoy, A.: The effect of cod liver oil and corn oil on platelets and vessel wall in man. Thromb. Haemostasis *46:* 604–611 (1981).

10 Darcet, P.; Driss, F.; Mendy, F.; Delhaye, N.: Exploration du métabolisme des acides gras des lipidex totaux plasmatiques et de l'agrégation plaquettaire d'une population d'hommes âgés à l'aide d'une alimentation enrichie en acide linolénique. Annls Nutr. Aliment. *34:* 277–290 (1980).

F. Driss, MD, Centre de Gérontologie, 49, rue Mirabeau, F–75016 Paris (France)

Wld Rev. Nutr. Diet., vol. 43, pp. 174–178 (Karger, Basel 1984)

Valproate-Induced Hyperammonemia: Role of Diet

C. Marescaux[a], *J.M. Warter*[a], *L. Rumbach*[a], *G. Micheletti*[a], *G. Chabrier*[b], *M. Imler*[b]

[a] Neurophysiopathology Research Group (Prof. *D. Kurtz*), Neurological Clinic, City Hospital, Strasbourg; [b] Internal Medicine Service (Prof. *M. Imler*), Hautepierre Hospital, Strasbourg, France

Introduction

Sodium valproate (VPA) (Dépakine®) always induces an arterial hyperammonemia [3, 4, 6] starting in the minutes following the first dose of VPA p.o. or i.v., and persisting during chronic treatment with the drug. Hepatic tests and acid-base factors remain normal. In the present work, we investigate the links between diet and the VPA-induced arterial hyperammonemia.

Material and Methods

The subjects were consenting epileptics, and healthy volunteers, members of the medical team. VPA was given p.o. in the form of 500 mg enterally absorbed tablets of Dépakine, and i.v., 400 mg injectable doses of LCG 211 17 (Labaz Laboratories). The standard diet consisted of a 7-a.m. breakfast, 485 kcal (9 g proteins, 18 g lipids, 72 g carbohydrates), a 1-p.m. lunch, 685 kcal (30 g proteins, 21 g lipids, 94 g carbohydrates) and a 7-p.m. supper, 765 kcal (31 g proteins, 28 g lipids, 97 g carbohydrates).

Blood was withdrawn via an indwelling catheter from the left radial artery. NH_4^+ concentration was measured by a colorimetric method on 50 µl whole blood [1], and the results expressed as µmol per liter (normal values, $\overline{X} \pm 2\,SD$, 28 ± 12 µmol/l). VPA was measured by gas chromatography and the results expressed in mg per liter of plasma.

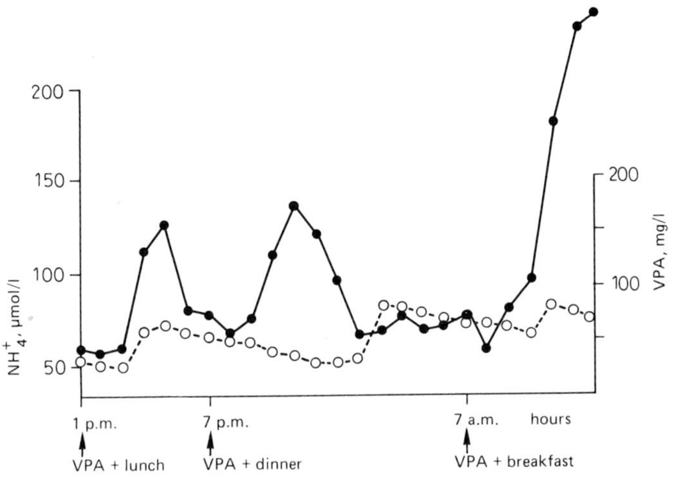

Fig. 1. Arterial ammonium concentrations vs time over a 1-day period in a patient treated for more than 1 year with VPA, 20 mg/kg/day in 3 doses, and phenobarbital, 2 mg/kg/day in 2 doses. ● = [NH_4^+], µmol/l blood; ○ = VPA, mg/l plasma.

Results

The arterial ammonemia, measured hourly on epileptics treated for over 1 year with VPA alone or in association with other anti-epileptics, was elevated and varied during the course of the day. The hyperammonemia was higher when VPA was given with other anti-epileptics, notably phenobarbital. The [NH_4^+] variations were not correlated with plasma VPA variations. Meals accentuated the hyperammonemia (fig. 1).

In order to examine the role of diet, hourly measurements were made on healthy volunteers after a single dose of VPA. A standard lunch eaten at a different time from the oral or intravenous absorption of VPA 15–25 mg/kg caused a notable increase of systemic hyperammonemia. The peak of [NH_4^+] occurred 1 h after the meal and subsided after 3 or 4 h (fig. 2). After the simultaneous absorption of a standard meal and VPA 15- to 25 mg/kg p.o., the ammonemia rose slowly in parallel with plasma VPA. [NH_4^+] did not then peak sharply, and VPA increased more slowly than in a fasting subject.

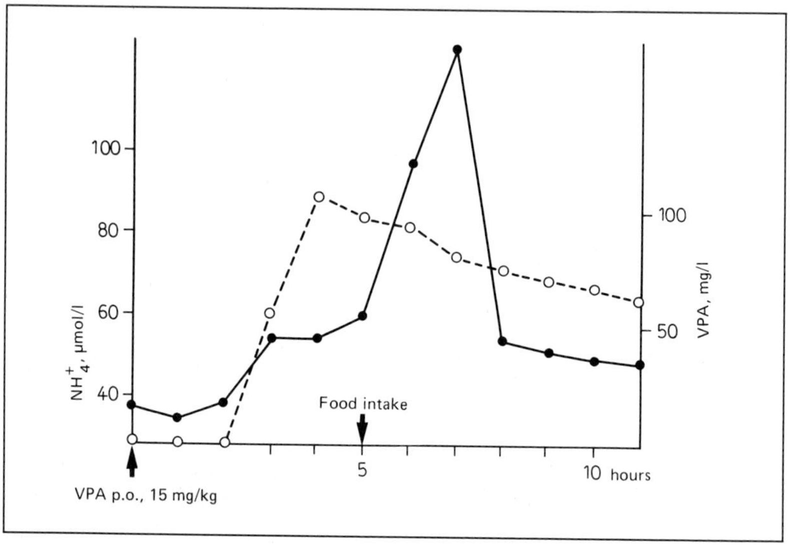

Fig. 2. Arterial [NH_4^+] vs time after absorption of VPA 15 mg/kg p.o. in fasting subject. Meal, 685 kcal. Symbols as in figure 1.

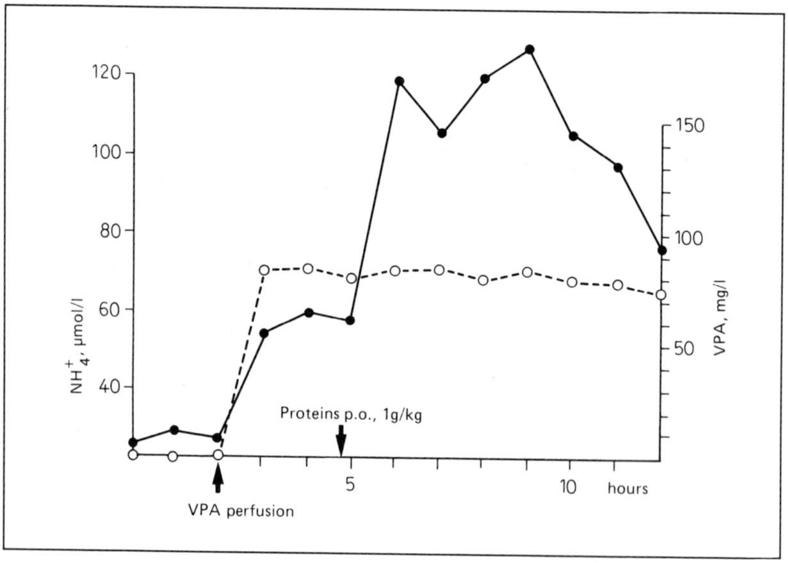

Fig. 3. Arterial [NH_4^+] vs time in subject under constant VPA perfusion. Protein, 1 g/kg, was absorbed 3 h after perfusion began. Symbols as in figure 1.

At an 8-day interval, 2 healthy volunteers ate a protein meal (1 g/kg) or a lipid meal (1 g/kg), while plasma VPA was maintained between 80 and 100 mg/l by a constant flow perfusion. The lipid meal did not modify the ammonemia. The protein meal, however, induced peaks of ammonemia independent of the plasma VPA levels (fig. 3).

Discussion

Because of the preponderant role played by the liver in ammonia metabolism, and the existence of rare hepatotoxic complications due to VPA, a sometimes mortal toxic hepatitis [5], it was logical to suppose that VPA-induced hyperammonemia was of hepatic origin. However, it has been shown in humans and rats that the hyperammonemia induced by treatment with VPA alone is of renal origin, the ammonia detoxification capacities of the liver remaining normal [7, 8]. Our present findings, in particular the observation of an accentuated hyperammonemia after a protein-rich meal, do not contradict other recent findings. *Imler* et al. [2] have further shown in the normal rat that the hyperammonemia induced by a high-protein regime is also of renal origin.

In conclusion, an isolated hyperammonemia is a constant metabolic consequence of treatments by VPA, and is accentuated by protein absorption. It depends on physiopathological mechanisms different from those underlying the hepatotoxic complications due to VPA.

References

1 Imler, M.; Frick, A.; Schlienger, J.L.; Stahl, A.: An automated microassay for blood ammonia. J. clin. chem. Biochem. *17:* 247–250 (1979).

2 Imler, M.; Schlienger, J.L.; Chabrier, G.; Comte, F.: Origine rénale de l'hyperammoniémie induite par un régime hyperprotidique chez le rat normal ou porteur d'une stricture portale. Gastroentérol. clin. biol. *6:* 22A (1982).

3 Marescaux, C.; Warter, J.M.; Laroye, M.; Rumbach, L.; Micheletti, G.; Koehl, C.; Imler, M.; Kurtz, D.: Le valproate de sodium: une drogue hyperammoniémiante. Etude chez l'épileptique et chez le volontaire sain. J. neurol. Sci. *58:* 195–209 (1983).

4 Murphy, J.V.; Marquardt, K.: Asymptomatic hyperammonemia in patients receiving valproic acid. Archs Neurol., Chicago *39:* 591–592 (1982).

5 Rothner, A.D.: Valproic acid: a review of 23 fatal cases. Ann. Neurol. *10:* 287 (1981).

6 Warter, J.M.; Marescaux, C.; Rumbach, L.; Galmiche, J.; Micheletti, G.; Koehl, C.; Imler, M.: L'hyperammoniémie isolée, une conséquence fréquente des traitements par le valproate de sodium. Nouv. Presse méd. *10:* 3406–3407 (1981).
7 Warter, J.M.; Brandt, C.M.; Marescaux, C.; Laroye, M.; Rumbach, L.; Micheletti, G.; Chabrier, G.; Imler, M.: Rôle du foie et des reins dans l'hyperammoniémie induite chez l'homme par le valproate de sodium seul ou associé au phénobarbital. J. Méd. Strasbourg *13:* 783–785 (1982).
8 Warter, J.M.; Imler, M.; Marescaux, C.; Chabrier, C.; Rumbach, L.; Micheletti, G.; Krieger, J.: Sodium valproate-induced hyperammonemia in the rat: role of the kidney. Eur. J. Pharmacol. *87:* 177–182 (1983).

C. Marescaux, MD, Neurophysiopathology Research (Prof. *D. Kurtz*), Neurological Clinic, City Hospital, F–67091 Strasbourg Cedex (France)

B. Drug Bioavailability and Metabolism

Wld Rev. Nutr. Diet., vol. 43, pp. 179–182 (Karger, Basel 1984)

Competition between Drugs and Nutrients for Specific Ligand Binding Sites on Human Serum Albumin[1]

E. Kiem, K.J. Fehske[2], *W.E. Müller*

Pharmakologisches Institut der Universität Mainz, Mainz, FRG

Introduction

After introduction into the circulation most drugs are bound to the different blood constituents (cells and proteins) whereof serum albumin is most important. Today, we have a variety of evidence that the actual number of drug binding sites of human serum albumin (HSA) is rather small and that several nutrients but especially *L*-tryptophan and the free fatty acids do also bind to these sites. Accordingly, competition is very likely to take place [3, 6, 8]. On the other hand, since only three ligand binding sites of HSA (the indole and benzodiazepine site, the digitoxin site, and the warfarin and azapropazone area) are mainly involved in the HSA binding of most drugs, it seems possible to predict the effects of lipids on the plasma binding of drugs, if each of the binding sites is affected in a characteristic way. Accordingly, the present communication describes some experiments on the effects of palmitic and oleic acids (the two most important fatty acids in human plasma) [2] on the HSA and human plasma binding of several drugs specific for one of the three important ligand binding sites.

Materials and Methods

Drug binding to HSA and human plasma was investigated by equilibrium dialysis [4] but at 37 °C and using a Krebs-Ringer phosphate buffer, pH 7.4, for the protein-free side of the 1-ml dialysis cells. Preliminary

[1] Supported by a grant of the Deutsche Forschungsgemeinschaft.

[2] Present address: Cassella-Riedel Pharma GmbH, D–6500 Frankfurt, FRG.

experiments indicated that under these conditions all drugs investigated are bound to one high affinity site of HSA. The effects of fatty acids were studied at concentrations of 50 and 120 mg/100 ml (experiments with human plasma) or at lower concentrations but representing similar molar fatty acid/HSA ratios (e.g. 0.6, 3, 7) (experiments with solutions of cristalline HSA 36 μmol/l).

Table I. Inhibition of the binding of several drugs to human serum albumin and human plasma by palmitic and oleic acids

Competitor mg/100 ml	Free fraction, % ($\bar{x} \pm$ SEM, n = 6)				
	diazepam	flurbiprofen	azapropazone	warfarin	digitoxin
Human serum albumin (36 μmol/l)					
Palmitic acid					
0	33.2 ± 0.4	6.9 ± 0.2	14.8 ± 00.2	24.8 ± 00.1	32.1 ± 2.3
10	36.4 ± 0.6	6.5 ± 0.1	14.0 ± 00.4	23.8 ± 00.1	32.0 ± 1.7
50	47.5 ± 0.2**	5.0 ± 0.1**	11.6 ± 00.4**	17.6 ± 00.3**	30.7 ± 1.4
120	55.3 ± 0.6**	5.5 ± 0.1*	13.8 ± 00.3	16.3 ± 0.1**	36.7 ± 1.1
Oleic acid					
0	30.8 ± 0.2	7.2 ± 0.1	13.6 ± 0.4	24.0 ± 0.2	34.3 ± 0.2
10	33.3 ± 1.3	6.5 ± 0.1	12.7 ± 0.3	21.9 ± 0.4	36.7 ± 1.4
50	47.7 ± 0.3**	4.8 ± 0.1**	11.5 ± 0.2	16.2 ± 0.3**	32.1 ± 1.0
120	64.6 ± 1.5**	12.8 ± 0.7**	36.9 ± 1.8**	30.1 ± 1.8**	59.0 ± 1.1**
Human plasma					
Palmitic acid					
0	2.1 ± 0.1	4.5 ± 0.4	13.2 ± 1.0	3.4 ± 0.2	14.7 ± 0.7
50	5.2 ± 0.1**	5.2 ± 0.3	13.4 ± 0.7	2.3 ± 0.1**	15.7 ± 0.5
120	8.7 ± 0.3**	7.3 ± 0.3**	15.0 ± 0.2*	2.9 ± 0.1*	20.0 ± 0.6**
Oleic acid					
0	2.2 ± 0.2	4.7 ± 0.2	11.9 ± 0.5	3.3 ± 0.1	14.1 ± 0.4
50	4.8 ± 0.4**	5.6 ± 0.3	12.3 ± 0.5	2.7 ± 0.1**	16.1 ± 0.4*
120	8.7 ± 0.3**	7.5 ± 0.2**	13.5 ± 0.4**	2.9 ± 0.1*	19.6 ± 1.1**

For the experiments with HSA molar drug/protein ratios of 1.1 and fatty acid/HSA ratios similar to the plasma levels indicated were used. For the experiments with human plasma the fatty acid concentrations indicated and the following drug concentrations were used: diazepam = 2 μmol/l; flurbiprofen = 10 μmol/l; azapropazone = 220 μmol/l; warfarin = 10 μmol/l; digitoxin = 0.05 μmol/l.

* $p < 0.05$, ** $p < 0.01$ when compared with controls [from ref. 5].

Results and Discussion

While cholesterol at concentrations relative (molar ratio to HSA) to plasma levels of 5 and 25 mg/100 ml did not alter the binding of all drugs indicated in table I to HSA, palmitic and oleic acids profoundly affect the binding of all drugs investigated, each specific for one of the three important ligand binding sites of HSA (see the free fractions without and in the presence of both fatty acids in table I).

Indole and Benzodiazepine Binding Site. Both fatty acids potently inhibit the binding of diazepam to this site either in the case of HSA or for human plasma. On the other hand, the binding of flurbiprofen to HSA, which is also associated with this site [4], is enhanced by medium concentrations of both fatty acids and is reduced only by high concentrations of oleic acid but not of palmitic acid. By contrast, both fatty acids at high concentrations inhibit the binding of flurbiprofen to human plasma.

Warfarin and Azapropazone Binding Area. Similar to previous reports [1, 7], drug binding to this site of HSA can be influenced by fatty acids in a two-phasic pattern. Both fatty acids enhance the HSA binding of warfarin and azapropazone to this site at medium concentrations, but only oleic acid decreases the binding of both drugs when added at high concentrations (corresponding to a molar ratio of about 7). However, using human plasma, only a small but significant decrease of the binding of azapropazone is observed for both fatty acids, while the binding of warfarin is significantly enhanced under similar conditions.

Digitoxin Binding Site. Both fatty acids strongly inhibit the binding of digitoxin to this site, an effect which can be seen for HSA as well as for human plasma.

In conclusion, the findings reported indicate that very distinct changes of the HSA binding of various drugs can be observed in the presence of physiological and pathological concentrations of palmitic and oleic acids. But more important, the effects observed for both fatty acids are not always similar for drugs bound to the same ligand binding site of HSA. While this observation was to some extent expected for the large warfarin and azapropazone binding area [4], it was quite unexpected for the indole and benzodiazepine binding site. Thus, it might become more difficult than originally thought to predict changes of the plasma binding of drugs due to pathological or nutrition-induced changes of the plasma levels of free fatty acids, even when the binding site(s) of the drugs on the HSA molecule are known.

References

1 Birkett, D.J.; Myers, S.P.; Sudlow, G.: Effects of fatty acids on two drug binding sites on human serum albumin. Molec. Pharmacol. *13:* 987–992 (1977).

2 Colombo, R.; Pinelli, A.: Effect of in vivo increase of free fatty acids on human plasma protein binding of furosemide. Pharmacology *25:* 73–81 (1982).

3 Fehske, K.J.; Müller, W.E.; Wollert, U.: The location of drug binding sites in human serum albumin. Biochem. Pharmacol. *30:* 687–692 (1981).

4 Fehske, K.J.; Schläfer, U.; Wollert, U.; Müller, W.E.: Characterization of an important drug binding area on human serum albumin including the high-affinity binding sites of warfarin and azapropazone. Molec. Pharmacol. *21:* 387–393 (1982).

5 Kiem, E.; Fehske, K.J.; Müller, W.E.: The effects of endogenous inhibitors on specific ligand binding sites of HSA (in preparation, 1983).

6 Kragh-Hansen, U.: Molecular aspects of ligand binding to serum albumin. Pharmacol. Rev. *33:* 17–53 (1981).

7 Müller, W.E.: The use of 8-anilino-1-naphthalenesulfonic acid as a reporter group molecule for circular dichroism and fluorescence measurements. The effects of stearic acid and sodium dodecylsulfate on the conformation of bovine and human serum albumin. Hoppe-Seyler's Z. physiol. Chem. *357:* 1487–1494 (1976).

8 Müller, W.E.; Wollert, U.: Human serum albumin as a 'silent receptor' for drugs and endogenous substances. Pharmacology *19:* 59–67 (1979).

PD Dr. Walter E. Müller, Psychopharmakologisches Labor,
Zentralinstitut für Seelische Gesundheit, J5, D-6800 Mannheim (FRG)

Wld Rev. Nutr. Diet., vol. 43, pp. 183–186 (Karger, Basel 1984)

Effects of a Meal and Its Composition on the Bioavailability of Betaxolol Administered Orally to Healthy Subjects

J.F. Thiercelin, G. Bianchetti, J. Larribaud, J. Ganansia, C. Deves, S. Trocherie, C. Abriol, P.L. Morselli

Lers-Synthelabo, Clinical Research Department, Paris, France

Introduction

The influence of food on the rate and extent of bioavailability of several adrenergic β-blocking agents has already been extensively studied. This is due to the fact that drugs belonging to this class have rather different pharmacokinetic properties. The bioavailabilities of propranolol, metoprolol and labetolol are increased by concomitant ingestion of food [2–4], although the contrary has been described for atenolol [5] and sotalol.

Thus, it seemed useful if not essential, to study the possible effect of food upon the gastrointestinal absorption of betaxolol, a new cardioselective β-blocker characterized by a long elimination half-life, a complete absorption and a very low hepatic first-pass effect.

Protocol

Subjects

9 healthy subjects of both sexes (7 males and 2 females), aged between 22 and 38 years and weighing between 49 and 84 kg, were selected for the study. These volunteers had taken no drugs during the 8 previous days nor throughout the duration of the trial.

Experimental Conditions

The study was performed according to an open cross-over design as 3 replicates of the same 3 × 3 Latin square. Treatments were separated by an interval of 1 week and consisted of 3 different experimental situations corresponding to: (A) fasting: no breakfast; (B) heavy 'English' breakfast: 673 cal composed of 26.8 g of protids, 31.7 g of lipids and 77.6 g of glucids; (C) light 'Continental' breakfast: 349 cal composed of 8.7 g of protids, 10.3 g of lipids, 75 g of glucids.

On each sequence, betaxolol was administered as a single 20-mg dose with 100 ml of water, 30 min after the breakfast, if any. A standard meal of 851 cal composed of 39 g of protids, 36 g of lipids and 80 g of glucids was given 4 h after drug intake. For each sequence, 5 ml of blood were drawn in heparinized tubes before drug intake and 0.5, 1, 1.5, 2, 3, 4, 5, 6, 8, 10, 12, 24, 28, 33, 48, 57 and 72 h after drug intake. Quantitation of betaxolol in blood was done by a gas chromatographic method described by *Bianchetti* et al. [1].

The statistical comparison of pharmacokinetic parameters (area under the curve, peak time, peak concentration, absorption and elimination half-lives were carried out by a two-way analysis of variance with subject and treatment as factors. The symmetrical confidence intervals were calculated by the method of *Westlake* [6].

Results

Mean pharmacokinetic results and statistical comparison between treatments are given in table I. Mean pharmacokinetic profiles obtained following treatment A, B and C are presented in figure 1. The symmetrical confidence intervals around the mean value of treatment A, taken as a reference, are given in table II. No statistically significant differences were detected for area under the curve ($AUC_0 \rightarrow \infty$, peak time (t_{max}), absorption

Table I. Mean (± SE) pharmacokinetic parameters of bataxolol after a single 20 mg oral dose was given in three different experimental conditions (n = 9)

Breakfast	t_{max} h	C_{max} ng/ml	$t_{1/2\alpha}$ h	$t_{1/2\beta}$ h	$AUC_0 \rightarrow \infty$ $ng \cdot h \cdot ml^{-1}$
A – Fasting	4.1±0.4	41±2.3	1.0±0.3	14.8±0.7	942±55
B – English	4.5±0.5	47±3.9	1.0±0.1	14.3±1.0	1,046±86
C – Continental	4.2±0.3	40±1.9	0.8±0.1	14.7±0.8	953±58
Statistical significance	n.s.	$p < 0.05$	n.s.	n.s.	n.s.

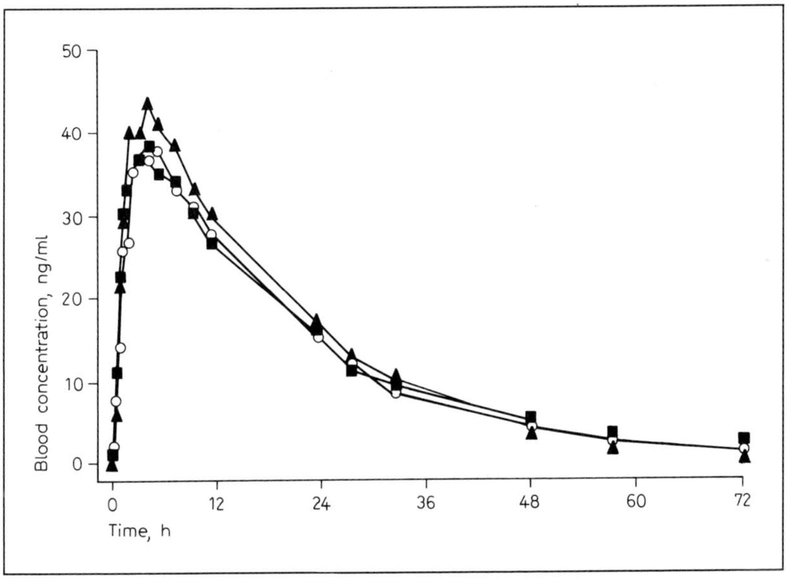

Fig. 1. Mean blood concentration-time profiles resulting from single doses of 20 mg of betaxolol given to 9 subjects in a fasting state (■), or after an English (▲) or Continental (○) breakfast.

Table II. Symmetrical confidence intervals (p = 0.95) of some pharmacokinetic parameters of betaxolol after a single 20 mg oral dose in three different experimental conditions. Fasting is taken as the reference condition

Parameters	English breakfast B	Fasting (reference) A	Continental breakfast C
$AUC_{0 \rightarrow \infty}$	758–1,126* (Δ = 19.6%)	942	842–1,042 (Δ = 10.6%)
C_{max}	30.9–51.9 (Δ = 24.6%)	41	35.9–46.1 (Δ = 12.5%)
t_{max}	2.67–5.45 (Δ = 34.1%)	4.1	2.73–5.38 (Δ = 29.0%)
$T_{1/2\beta}$	13.1–16.4 (Δ = 11.2)	14.8	13.3–16.24 (Δ = 9.8)

* Confidence interval limits (p = 0.95; n = 9).
** Confidence interval expressed as a percentage of the reference value.

half-life ($t_{1/2\alpha}$) and elimination half-life ($t_{1/2\beta}$). Only the maximum concentration (C_{max}) was significantly ($p < 0.05$) increased after the 'English' type breakfast. However, this 15% increase is lying within the commonly admitted bounds of 25% around the mean C_{max} for treatment A and is therefore not likely to have any clinical relevance.

Discussion

The lack of effect of food on the bioavailability of betaxolol is in good agreement with the pharmacokinetic characteristics of this drug. The absence of first-pass effect is probably the reason why this new drug is not influenced by variations in hepatic blood flow and by the presence of compounds (food or drug) which are highly extracted by the liver.

From these experimental findings, it is possible to draw some practical conclusions: (1) Since the ingestion and composition of meals did not affect the bioavailability of betaxolol, it should be possible to administer the drug either before, during or after meals. This will obviously provide a degree of flexibility in prescribing the drug. (2) The absence of food-related effects on the absorption of betaxolol is an important factor in explaining the low intra- and inter-variability observed with this drug. This feature should facilitate the task of the clinician when adjusting the dose to a patient.

References

1 Bianchetti, G.; et al.: Sensitive gas-chromatographic method for the determination in blood and urine of SL 75 212, a new β_1-adrenoreceptor blocking agent. J. Chromatogr., biomed. Appl. *176:* 134–139 (1979).
2 Mantyla, R.; et al.: Effect of food on the bioavailability of labetolol. Br. J. clin. Pharmacol. *9:* 435–437 (1980).
3 Melander, A.; et al.: Enhancement of bioavailability of propranolol and metoprolol by food. Clin. Pharmacol. Ther. *22:* 108–112 (1977).
4 Melander, A.; et al.: Influence of food on the bioavailability of drugs. Clin. Pharmacokinet. *3:* 337–351 (1978).
5 Malander, A.; et al.: Food induced reduction in bioavailability of atenolol. Eur. J. clin. Pharmacol. *16:* 327–330 (1979).
6 Westlake, W.J.: Symmetrical confidence intervals for bioequivalence trials. Biometrics *32:* 741–744 (1976).

J.E. Thiercelin, MD, Lers-Synthelabo, Clinical Research Department,
58, rue de la Glacière, F–75013 Paris (France)

Wld Rev. Nutr. Diet., vol. 43, pp. 187–191 (Karger, Basel 1984)

Influence of Dietary Purines on the Metabolism of Allopurinol in Man[1]

S. Reiter, W. Löffler, W. Gröbner, N. Zöllner

Medizinische Poliklinik der Universität München, München, FRG

Introduction

Allopurinol influences both purine and pyrimidine metabolism: it reduces the formation of uric acid by inhibition of xanthine oxidase and induces oroticaciduria by inhibition of orotidylic acid (OMP) decarboxylase. This influence considerably depends on the purine content of diet: when a purine-free diet is replaced by a diet rich in purines, the formation of uric acid is decreased to a much higher degree [3] and oroticaciduria is greatly diminished [4]. As the underlying mechanisms are still unknown we have performed nutrition experiments to prove a possible influence of dietary purines on the metabolism of allopurinol.

Methods

12 healthy students received a purine-free isoenergetic formula diet and 0.5–1 g allopurinol daily for 2 weeks. During the second week different purines were administered orally together with allopurinol in an equimolar or 1.5-fold increased dose (table I). In the 24-hour urines the concentrations of allopurinol and purine metabolites were determined by high pressure liquid chromatography (HPLC) on a Hewlett-Packard 1084B system with a Chrompack RP-8 column using an isocratic modification of the method of *Webster* et al. [2]. Urine samples were preseparated on small anion-exchange columns.

[1] These studies were supported by the Deutsche Forschungsgemeinschaft.

Table I. Influence of dietary purines on the formation of allopurinol-1-riboside

Subject	Daily dose of		Urinary excretion of allopurinol-1-riboside (% of total urinary excretion of allopurinol and its metabolites)		Increase of urinary purine metabolites (mmol/24 h) due to administration of dietary purines		
	purine mmol	allopurinol mg	purine-free period	administration of purines	hypoxanthine	xanthine	uric acid
1 Hypoxanthine	1×7.5	1×1,000	22.6	1.3	2.6	0.96	0.71
2 Hypoxanthine	1×7.5	1×675	12.4	1.2	2.2	1.08	0
3 Inosine	1×6.5	1×600	20	0.9	0.75	0.48	0
4 IMP	1×6.7	1×600	13	6	1.01	0.78	0.54
5 Adenine	1×8.3	1×750	11	0	2.93	1.37	0.17
6 Adenine	3×2.8	3×245	24.6	1.8	1.94	2.39	0
7 Adenosine	1×9.0	1×825	13	3	0.75	0.52	0.02
8 Adenosine	3×2.9	3×258	20.7	2.8	1.54	2.51	0
9 AMP	1×8.3	1×750	16	7	0.87	0.91	0.01
10 AMP	3×2.5	3×225	20.9	3	1.41	2.06	0.12
11 Guanosine	1×5.9	1×800	20	16	0.04	2.25	0.7
12 GMP	1×5.3	1×725	9	4	0.01	2.23	0.45

IMP = Inosine monophosphate; AMP = adenosine monophosphate; GMP = guanosine monophosphate.

Results and Discussion

During the purine-free period an average of 74% of the allopurinol dose was recovered in the urine, mostly as oxipurinol, which represented 61–74% of total urinary metabolites; unchanged allopurinol amounted to 9–20%; 9–25% consisted of the second major metabolite of allopurinol, allopurinol-1-riboside, a compound without an inhibitory effect on xanthine oxidase. The administration of dietary purines markedly decreased the excretion of allopurinol-1-riboside: in the centre part of table I the percentage of allopurinol-1-riboside excretion during the purine-free period as compared to the period of purine administration is listed for all experiments.

The administration of hypoxanthine, inosine, adenine, adenosine and AMP caused a strong decrease of allopurinol-1-riboside excretion; guanosine was the less effective compound. In an additional nutrition experiment it was demonstrated that this decrease of allopurinol-1-riboside excretion is due to an inhibition of its formation: in this experiment the 24-hour urines were collected in 5 periods of 4–8 h each to study the excretion pattern of allopurinol-1-riboside. Because the latter was not changed by a delayed intake of hypoxanthine 5 h after the administration of allopurinol, we conclude that dietary purines like hypoxanthine do not influence the renal excretion of allopurinol-1-riboside but inhibit its synthesis when taken simultaneously with allopurinol.

To clarify the mechanism by which dietary purines inhibit the formation of allopurinol-1-riboside we studied their metabolic fate: in the right part of table I the urinary metabolites derived from the administered purines in the presence of allopurinol are listed. There was no or only a small conversion of dietary purines to uric acid indicating that this metabolite does not contribute to the inhibition of allopurinol-1-riboside synthesis. Considering the data of the guanosine experiment where a large formation of xanthine corresponded to only a small decrease of allopurinol-1-riboside formation, it seems most likely that also xanthine has no influence on the synthesis of allopurinol-1-riboside. Therefore, hypoxanthine seems to be the only effective metabolite of the administered purines. Figure 1 demonstrates that there is indeed a significant reciprocal correlation between the formation of allopurinol-1-riboside and hypoxanthine, whereas the formation of xanthine, in this case due to the administration of guanosine, is not correlated to the synthesis of allopurinol-1-riboside.

A significant reciprocal correlation between hypoxanthine and allopurinol-1-riboside excretion or formation respectively was found in 10 out of

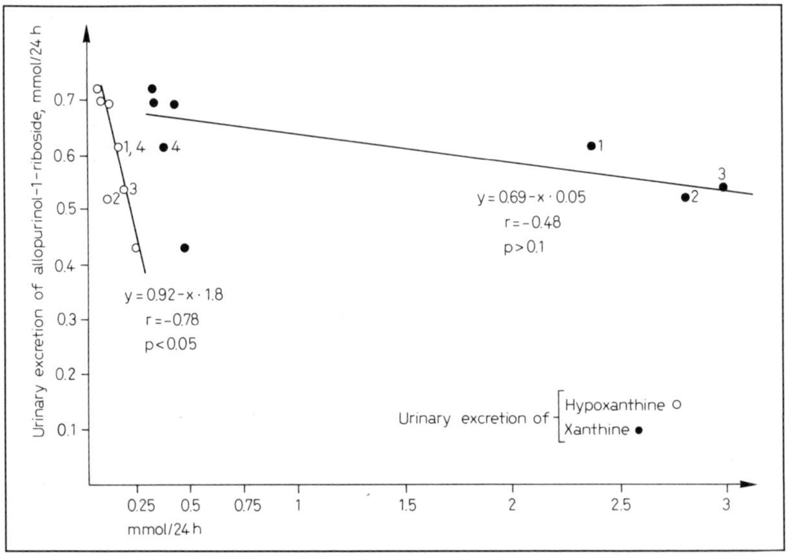

Fig. 1. Correlation between the formation of allopurinol-1-riboside and hypoxanthine or xanthine during the purine free period and during the administration of guanosine (points 1–3).

12 experiments ($p < 0.05$). There are two possible mechanisms by which hypoxanthine may inhibit the formation of allopurinol-1-riboside: the latter compound can be synthesized either directly by purine nucleoside phosphorylase (PNP) or indirectly via allopurinol-1-ribotide, a product of hypoxanthine guanine phosphoribosyltransferase (HGPRT); hypoxanthine serves as an excellent substrate for both enzymes. Since PNP functions in animal tissues primarily in the direction of nucleoside breakdown and we have recently found a large formation of allopurinol-1-riboside in a patient with a complete PNP-deficiency [1], we believe that the indirect biosynthesis of allopurinol-1-riboside via the nucleotide predominates in vivo. Consequently, we assume that hypoxanthine, derived from dietary purines in the presence of allopurinol, decreases the formation of allopurinol-1-riboside by competitive inhibition of the enzyme HGPRT.

The inhibition of allopurinol-1-riboside formation by dietary purines results in an elevated excretion of oxipurinol and unchanged allopurinol, the average urinary recovery of allopurinol and its metabolites being not influenced. This indicates a raised bioavailability of the drug because allopurinol-1-riboside has no inhibitory effect on xanthine oxidase.

References

1 Reiter, S.; Simmonds, H.A.; Webster, D.R.; Watson, A.R.: On the metabolism of allopurinol: formation of allopurinol-1-riboside in purine nucleoside phosphorylase deficiency. Biochem. Pharmac. *32:* 2167–2174 (1983).
2 Webster, D.R.; Simmonds, H.A.; Barry, D.M.J.; Becroft, D.M.O.: Pyrimidine and purine metabolites in ornithine carbamoyl transferase deficiency. J. inher. metab. Dis. *4:* 27–31 (1981).
3 Zöllner, N.; Gröbner, W.: Der unterschiedliche Einfluss von Allopurinol auf die endogene und exogene Uratquote. Eur. J. clin. Pharmacol. *3:* 56–58 (1970).
4 Zöllner, N.; Gröbner, W.: Influence of oral ribonucleic acid on oroticaciduria due to allopurinol administration. Z. ges. exp. Med. *156:* 317–319 (1971).

S. Reiter, MD, Medizinische Poliklinik der Universität München,
D–8000 München 2 (FRG)

C. Effect of Malnutrition on Drug Pharmacokinetics

Wld Rev. Nutr. Diet., vol. 43, pp. 192–197 (Karger, Basel 1984)

Steady-State Kinetics of Salicylic Acid in Undernutrition

R. Arunkumar Shastri

National Institute of Nutrition, Jamai-Osmania, Hyderabad, India

Introduction

There are a number of reports now to show that malnutrition in man alters drug kinetics [1–3]. With the information available to date, it may be stated that the influence of malnutrition in adults on drug metabolism is different from that in malnourished children [3, 4] thereby suggesting that the pathophysiology of adult malnutrition is probably different from that of childhood malnutrition, at least as far as pharmacokinetics is concerned. In spite of a large number of anti-inflammatory drugs now available, acetylsalicylic acid (ASA) continues to be the most widely used because of its efficacy, low toxicity and low cost [5]. ASA has a very short half-life and is immediately hydrolysed to salicylic acid (SA) in the body. Since there is no information on SA kinetics in undernourished adults, the study reported here was carried out to investigate the effect of malnutrition in adults on SA steady-state kinetics.

Materials and Methods

The subjects investigated were classified as well-nourished (n = 18) or undernourished (n = 17) based on their anthropometric index weight/height^2 $\times$ 100 (weight in kilograms, height in centimeters). Subjects with an index below 0.18 were classified as undernourished [6].

Three different daily doses of ASA were employed for the study, namely 30, 50 and 100 mg/kg body weight. ASA was administered in 4 equally divided doses at 8 a.m., 2 p.m., 8 p.m. and 2 a.m. until plasma steady-state concentrations were reached. Blood samples from subjects being investigated with the 30-mg/kg dose of ASA were obtained on two consecutive days at 8 a.m. just before the subsequent dose at the end of 48 and 72 h. The blood samples in the 50- and 100-mg/kg dose of ASA studies were obtained on 3 consecutive days at 8 a.m. just before the subsequent dose at the end of 96, 120 and 144 h.

24 urinary collections of the subjects were made under toluene for the entire duration of the studies. Plasma SA was measured by a modification of Brodie's method [7]. pH measurements were made on all samples of urine on a pH meter routinely standardized with buffer solutions of pH 4.0 and 8.0. Serum albumin concentrations were determined by the biuret method [8]. Plasma protein binding of SA was determined by ultrafiltration of the plasma obtained from subjects receiving 100 mg/kg body weight of ASA.

Clearance of total SA (Cl_T) was calculated by the formula $Cl_T = R/C_p$, where R represents the dose in mg per unit time and C_p the steady-state plasma concentration of SA. Unbound clearance (Clu) was calculated using the equation $Clu = \frac{R}{Cu}$, where Cu represents the concentration of unbound SA in plasma at steady state. For calculations of clearance it was assumed that the absorption of ASA was complete in all the subjects. Secondly, the SA concentrations used in the calculations were C_{min} plasma concentrations and not the average plasma concentrations at steady state. The clearance values obtained are, therefore, referred to as the apparent clearance of SA. Statistical analyses were carried out using the Student's t-test.

Results

The results of the studies with all the three different doses are presented in tables I–III. Both the anthropometric indices and serum albumin concentrations were significantly lower in the undernourished subjects as compared to the well-nourished. However, the mean plasma SA concentrations were similar in the two groups, irrespective of the dose of ASA employed. In the 100-mg/kg body weight ASA study, the plasma protein binding of SA was similar in the two groups investigated (table III).

There were no significant differences in the clearance of total SA, between the groups of well-nourished and undernourished subjects, irre-

Table I. Anthropometric index, serum albumin, plasma concentrations and apparent clearance of salicylic acid (aspirin dose 30 mg/kg)

Group	Weight/height^2 × 100	Serum albumin g/l	Plasma concentrations, mg/100 ml		Clearance ml/h/kg	Urinary pH
			48 h	72 h		
Well-nourished (8)	0.21 ± 0.008	39.8 ± 0.08	4.8 ± 0.58	4.7 ± 1.2	31.82 ± 5.771	6.24 ± 0.07
Undernourished (6)	0.16 ± 0.002*	30.7 ± 0.12*	4.3 ± 0.89	3.7 ± 0.78	37.13 ± 8.422	6.12 ± 0.12

Values are means ± SE. Figures in parentheses indicate number of observations. * $p < 0.001$.

Table II. Anthropometric index, serum albumin, plasma concentrations and apparent clearance of salicylic acid (aspirin dose 50 mg/kg)

Group	Weight/height^2 × 100	Serum albumin g/l	Plasma concentrations, mg/100 ml			Clearance ml/h/kg	Urine pH
			96 h	120 h	144 h		
Well-nourished (6)	0.19 ± 0.006	39.4 ± 0.13	8.32 ± 1.479	7.84 ± 1.032	7.19 ± 1.348	28.93 ± 4.075	6.17 ± 0.171
Undernourished (6)	0.15 ± 0.013*	31.7 ± 0.19*	7.36 ± 0.934	8.01 ± 0.328	7.62 ± 0.408	28.09 ± 1.361	6.09 ± 0.158

Values are means ± SE. Figures in parentheses indicate number of observations. * $p < 0.05$.

Table III. Anthropometric index, serum albumin, plasma concentrations and apparent clearance of salicylic acid (aspirin dose 100 mg/kg)

Group	Weight/ height^2 × 100	Serum albumin g/l	Plasma concentrations, mg/100 ml			Clearance of total drug ml/h/kg, Cl_T	Clearance of unbound drug ml/h/kg, Clu	Plasma protein binding, %	Urinary pH
			96 h	120 h	144 h				
Well-nourished (6)	0.19 ± 0.005	37.9 ± 0.125	35.14 ± 4.740	36.32 ± 5.862	36.51 ± 6.266	10.56 ± 1.195	24.24 ± 3.031	57.7 ± 4.69	5.98 ± 0.080
Under-nourished (5)	0.15 ± 0.005*	24.8 ± 0.221*	34.09 ± 2.676	34.92 ± 1.164	36.04 ± 2.298	12.07 ± 0.464	28.13 ± 2.355	56.7 ± 4.97	6.02 ± 0.095

Values are means ± SE. Figures in parentheses indicate number of observations. * $p < 0.001$.

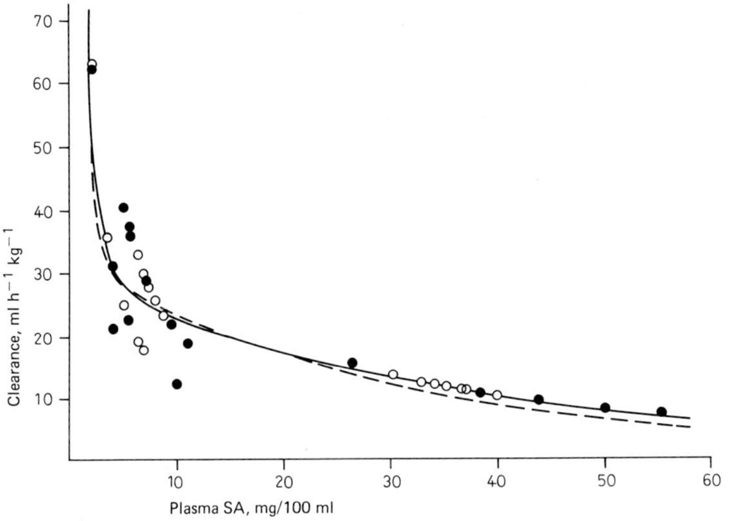

Fig. 1. Apparent clearance of SA plotted against plasma concentrations in well-nourished (○) and undernourished (●) subjects. Both groups exhibit a similar plasma concentration-dependent clearance of SA.

Table IV. Total apparent clearance of salicylate in the groups studied (ml/h/kg)

Dose of ASA mg/kg	Groups	
	well-nourished	undernourished
30	31.82 ± 5.771 (7)	37.13 ± 8.422 (6)
50	28.93 ± 4.075 (6)	28.09 ± 1.361 (6)
100	10.56 ± 1.195 (6)[a, b]	12.07 ± 0.464 (6)[a, c]

Values are means ± SE. Figures in parentheses indicate number of observations.
[a] $p < 0.01$ compared with the 30-mg/kg dose.
[b] $p < 0.02$ compared with the 50-mg/kg dose.
[c] $p < 0.05$ compared with the 50-mg/kg dose.

spective of the dose of ASA employed (tables I–III). It was, however, observed that as the dose of ASA was increased the clearance of total SA decreased and was significantly lower with the 100-mg/kg body weight dose in both well-nourished and undernourished subjects as compared to the clearances with 30 and 50 mg/kg body weight of ASA (table IV, fig. 1). The clearance of unbound SA in the undernourished group which received 100 mg/kg body weight of ASA was similar to that seen in the well-nourished (table III).

Discussion

The most important observation made in the present study is that the steady-state plasma concentrations of SA are unaltered and therefore the metabolism of SA in undernourished adults is similar to that in the well-nourished. There are several reports to indicate that the free fraction of SA is increased in hypoalbuminaemia [9, 10]. Earlier, our own studies with tetracycline, sulphadiazine and sulphafurazole have shown that the binding of these drugs to plasma proteins is significantly reduced in malnourished subjects [1, 2, 11]. It is, therefore, not clear why in the study reported here the free fractions of SA in plasma in undernourished subjects were similar to those seen in the well-nourished in spite of significant hypoalbuminaemia. *Anton and Corey* [12] have hypothesised, based on their observations on plasma protein binding of sulphonamides in hypoalbuminaemic patients that proteins which are not normally important for binding drugs in plasma may become important in certain disease states.

The clearance of total SA was found to decrease as the dose of ASA was increased in both the groups of subjects. The significant decrease observed in clearance of SA when the dose was increased to 100 mg/kg body weight is suggestive of a dose-dependent clearance of SA and is in agreement with that reported earlier by *Furst* et al. [13] who also found a dose-dependent decrease in the clearance of SA, but more so in the case of unbound SA.

In keeping with the observation that neither the steady-state levels nor the plasma protein binding of SA were unaltered in undernutrition, the clearances of total SA as well as unbound SA were similar in well-nourished and undernourished subjects. It may, therefore, be concluded that steady-state kinetics of SA are not altered in adults suffering from undernutrition and, therefore, no modification of dosage schedule would be necessary when treating them with ASA.

Acknowledgements

The author is presently recipient of a fellowship granted by the Foundation for Medical Research, Paris, at the Département de Pharmacologie, Faculté de Médecine de Créteil, Université de Paris XII, Créteil, France.

The author would like to thank Dr. *P.G. Tulpule,* Director, National Institute of Nutrition, Hyderabad, for his keen interest in the study. The useful discussions with and the help rendered by Prof. *J.P. Tillement* and Mr. *J. Barre* during the preparation of the manuscript are deeply appreciated.

References

1 Shastri, R.A.; Krishnaswamy, K.: Under nutrition and tetracycline half-life. Clinica chim. Acta *66:* 157–164 (1976).
2 Shastri, R.A.; Krishnaswamy, K.: Metabolism of sulphadiazine in malnutrition. Br. J. clin. Pharmacol. *7:* 69–73 (1979).
3 Buchanan, N.; Eyeberg, C.; Davis, M.D.: Isoniazid pharmacokinetics in kwashiorkor. S. Afr. med. J. *56:* 299–300 (1979).
4 Shastri, R.A.: Undernourished adults and acetylation phenotype. Int. J. clin. Pharm. Ther. Tox. *20:* 194–196 (1982).
5 Simon, L.S.; Mills, J.A.: Drug therapy: non steroidal anti-inflammatory drugs. New Engl. J. Med. *302:* 1179–1185 (1980).
6 Jayarao, K.S.; Mukerjee, N.R.; Rao, K.V.: A survey of diabetes mellitus in a rural population in India. Diabetes *21:* 1192–1196 (1972).
7 Routh, J.I.; Dryer, R.L.: Salicylate; in Seligson, Standard methods of clinical chemistry, vol. 3 (Academic Press, New York 1961).
8 Gornall, A.G.; Bardawill, L.J.; David, M.M.: Determination of serum proteins by means of the biuret reaction. J. biol. Chem. *177:* 751–766 (1949).
9 Borga, O.; Odar-Cederlof, I.; Ringberger, V.I.; Norlin, A.: Protein binding of salicylate in uraemic and normal plasma. Clin. Pharmacol. Ther. *20:* 464–475 (1976)
10 Wallace, S.; Brodie, M.J.: Decreased drug binding in serum from patients with chronic hepatic disease. Eur. J. clin. Pharmacol. *9:* 429–432 (1976).
11 Shastri, R.A.: Kinetics of sulphafurazole in undernutrition. Br. J. clin. Pharmacol. *10:* 499–502 (1980).
12 Anton, A.A.; Corey, W.T.: Protein binding of sulfonamides. Acta pharmac. tox. *29:* suppl. 3, pp. 134–150 (1971).
13 Furst, D.E.; Tozer, T.N.; Melmon, K.L.: Salicylate clearance, the resultant of protein binding and metabolism. Clin. Pharmacol. Ther. *26:* 380–389 (1979).

Dr. R.A. Shastri, MD, Département de Pharmacologie,
Faculté de Médecine de Créteil, Université de Paris XII,
8, rue du Général-Sarrail, F–94010 Créteil (France)

Subject Index